Pre-Writing

Skill Starters for Motor Development

Revised

by Marsha Dunn Klein, M.Ed., OTR/L

Illustrations drawn under contract by
Corwyn Zimbleman

Therapy Skill Builders®
a division of
The Psychological Corporation
555 Academic Court
San Antonio, Texas 78204-2498
1-800-228-0752

Reproducing Pages from This Book

As described below, some of the pages in this book may be reproduced for instructional or administrative use (not for resale). To protect your book, make a photocopy of each reproducible page. Then use that copy as a master for photocopying.

The Learning Curve Design is a registered trademark of The Psychological Corporation.

Copyright © 1982, 1990 by

Therapy Skill Builders®
a division of
The Psychological Corporation
555 Academic Court
San Antonio, Texas 78204-2498
1-800-228-0752

All rights reserved. No part of this publication may be reproduced or transmitted in any form or by any means, electronic or mechanical, including photocopying and recording, or by any information storage and retrieval system, without written permission from the publisher.

Permission is hereby granted to reproduce activity pages, checklists, and recordkeeping forms in this publication in complete pages, with the copyright notice, for administrative or instructional use and not for resale.

The Learning Curve Design and *Therapy Skill Builders* are registered trademarks of The Psychological Corporation.

ISBN 0761620893

10 11 12 A B C D E

Printed in the United States of America.

Please visit our Web site at www.PsychCorp.com. Please go to www.psychcorp.com/catg/pdf/survey.pdf to comment on this or any of our products. Your feedback is important to us.

About the Author

After receiving the B.S. degree in Occupational Therapy from Sargent College of Allied Health Professions at Boston University and the Master's degree in Education from the University of Arizona, **Marsha Dunn Klein** worked with developmentally disabled and physically handicapped persons at the Arizona Training Program for five years. In 1980 she received the Neurodevelopmental Treatment Certificate in pediatrics. Currently she is in private practice as a pediatric therapist in Tucson, Arizona.

Contents

Introduction 1

Objectives 3

1 Prerequisite Skills for Success in Pre-Writing Activities 5
Five Principles of Motor Skill Development 5
Nine Prerequisites for Learning to Write 6

2 Developmental Stages in Acquiring Pre-Writing Skills 11
Initial Stages 11
Imitation and Copying 14
Overview of Pre-Writing Developmental Stages 22
Checklist for Assessing Pre-Writing Developmental Skills
    (reproducible form) 23

3 Developmental Stages in Learning to Color 25
Picture Area 26
Checklist for Assessing Ability to Color a Picture Area
    (reproducible form) 30
Stroke Control 31
Checklist for Assessing Ability to Control Stroke
    (reproducible form) 35
Use of Color 36
Checklist for Assessing Ability to Use Color
    (reproducible form) 37
Overview of Coloring Skills Development 38

4 Choosing Appropriate Pre-Writing Materials 39
Sensory Media 40
Proprioceptive Media 42
Vestibular Media 42
Recipes for Finger Paint 44

5 Adaptive Techniques for Problem Areas 45
Balance 45
Poor Stability 51
Confusion about Dominance 55

    Poor Lead-Assist Hand Activity..56
    Poor Grasp and Control of the Writing Tool................................ 57
    Difficulty in Moving from an Immature to a Mature Grasp.......... 62
    Poor Attention Span..64
    Poor Imitation Skills... 66
    Limited Vision.. 67
    Inability to Use Hands... 69

6 Adaptive Pre-Writing Equipment..................................71
    Distributors' Addresses... 82

7 Movement and Pre-Writing Skills..............................83

8 Pre-Writing Activities... 89
    Pre-Writing Activity (reproducible form)....................................104

9 Weekly Activity Planning.. 105
    Weekly Pre-Writing Activity Plan (reproducible form).............. 106

10 Planning an Individual Pre-Writing Program............ 109
    Individual Pre-Writing Program (reproducible form)................. 111

Post-Test..112

Readings...119

Introduction

Writing is a complicated perceptual/motor/cognitive skill. Think about all the preparatory activities children take part in before kindergarten and first grade so they will be ready for the teacher's writing instruction. The skills necessary to learn to write are called *pre-writing skills*.

This workbook is for parents, preschool teachers, special education teachers, therapists—and anyone else who is interested in teaching pre-writing skills. First we will look at the prerequisite abilities. Then we will examine the developmental stages children go through in acquiring those skills. We will see that coloring pictures teaches important skills. The control that children learn in coloring complements the control they are learning simultaneously in pre-writing activities.

Checklists are provided for evaluating children's pre-writing and coloring skills. Appropriate materials and tools are discussed, and some classroom activities are presented. Finally, guidelines are given for creating individual pre-writing programs and preparing a week's series of activities that help children to develop a particular skill.

The workbook is designed to be a tool for independent study. It begins by listing specific objectives, and it ends with a test that helps you assess what you have learned. Periodic probes help you to reinforce the information you have just read. Throughout, illustrations help you to visualize the activities being discussed.

Objectives

By the end of this workbook, you will be able to:

1. List nine skills necessary before beginning pre-writing activities.
2. Explain the difference between imitation and copying.
3. List the developmental sequence of acquiring pre-writing skills.
4. Describe the developmental sequence of learning to color a picture area.
5. Describe the developmental stages of learning stroke control in coloring.
6. Describe the developmental sequence of learning to use color.
7. Name two visual media that can be used in choosing pre-writing materials.
8. Name two tactile media that can be used in choosing pre-writing materials.
9. Name two olfactory media that can be used in choosing pre-writing materials.
10. Name two auditory media that can be used in choosing pre-writing materials.
11. Name two gustatory media that can be used in choosing pre-writing materials.
12. Name two proprioceptive media that can be used in choosing pre-writing materials.
13. Describe a stable seating option, tell when it is used, and name two stable seating options.
14. Describe a practice seating option, tell when it is used, and name five practice seating options.
15. Name five things that can be done to improve stability for pre-writing functions.
16. Describe how the use of tools influences development of hand dominance.
17. Name an activity that can assist the writer who has poor two-hand usage.
18. For each of the following categories, list a pre-writing activity that does not require usual writing tools: gross motor activities; fine motor activities; sensory activities; daily living activities.

19. Name two options that may assist in moving from an immature to a mature grasp.

20. List six ways to vary sensory aspects of the pre-writing task to help students improve their attention span.

21. Describe two ways to increase sensory information in an imitation activity.

22. Describe two ways to provide sensory information for children with limited vision.

23. Name two ways for students to practice pre-writing concepts when they do not have functional use of their hands.

24. List seven types of adaptive equipment that can be used in teaching pre-writing skills, and explain the purpose of each.

25. List seven movement activities that can be used to reinforce shapes important for pre-writing skills.

26. List five classroom activities that can be used to teach pre-writing skills.

27. Describe how the same pre-writing activity can be taught in a variety of ways.

28. Describe how to incorporate information about pre-writing skills into an Individual Pre-Writing Program.

1 Prerequisite Skills for Success in Pre-Writing Activities

Before we analyze the prerequisite skills necessary to ensure success in pre-writing, we must understand how children normally acquire new motor skills.

Five Principles of Motor Skill Development

Principle 1 Children develop motor skills in a *cephalo-caudal* direction. In other words, they develop control of movements in a head-to-toe direction. They learn head control and shoulder control before walking or fine motor skills are achieved.

Principle 2 Control of movements is gained in a *proximal-to-distal* direction. This means that children learn to control the joints closest to the body (proximal) before being able to control the joints farthest away from the body (distal). They learn to reach and control shoulder movement before achieving elbow, wrist, and finger control.

Principle 3 *Stability* must be achieved before mobility or controlled distal movements are possible. Infants gain control of their shoulders through the process of lying on the tummy and moving their weight from side to side and forward and backward. Control is further refined as the infant crawls and creeps on all fours. We know that stability is being developed because we can see the infant reaching in more and more controlled ways with arms held farther away from the midline. As the shoulders gain stability, the weight-bearing and weight-shifting activities in the elbows and wrists help to refine that more distal control. Now the child can sit and turn the forearms to play with toys in a palm-up or supinated position. As forearm skill is achieved, the child continues to practice grasping a variety of objects with different sizes and shapes from a variety of positions. Children eventually will hold objects in one side of their hands (mobile side) while they creep on the floor with weight on the other side of their hands (stable side).

Principle 4 First movements are "whole-body" movements. Later, the child learns to *disassociate*, or separate the movements of one particular part of the body. Young infants first "reach" with both arms, legs, eyes, and even the mouth! Gradually they learn to separate their movements so one arm, the legs, and the mouth can rest quietly while the other arm effectively reaches. In grasping, first the whole hand is used. All fingers do the same thing at the same time. Gradually, children learn to move the thumb separately and in opposition to the fingers and to use fingers separately for the refined demands of precise grasping.

Principle 5 Children must pay attention to survival issues first. If they are unbalanced and feel as if they may fall off the chair, they will put their attention to their seating rather than to the fine motor task being taught. If the child is hungry, sick, or uncomfortable, these sensations will require all the attention.

Nine Prerequisites for Learning to Write

With an understanding of these five principles, we are ready to look at some specific prerequisites to successful development of pre-writing skills. Some of these skills may be missing in children who have physical or sensorimotor difficulties. For these children, pre-writing instruction can be adapted in some of the ways presented later in this book.

Prerequisite 1 **Developmental Readiness**

Children go through various stages when they are learning to play and interact with their environment. One of the earliest stages can be called the sensory explorative stage, in which the body itself is the child's toy. In this stage, children learn how to move their body parts, to isolate reach and grasp, and to coordinate those skills with vision. Mouthing, reaching, grasping, dropping, shaking, banging, and throwing dominate this stage. At this stage, children are not ready to be given a crayon. Mouthing, dropping, and shaking are inappropriate behaviors to utilize with a crayon.

Gradually, interest turns to learning how toys work. Cause-and-effect toys are the most interesting at that stage. Children develop specific pushing, pulling, poking, turning, and rolling skills. They explore new toys by dumping them out and taking them apart. If a crayon is given at this stage, mouthing, banging, or throwing commonly are seen—so these children still are not ready.

Children then enter the constructive stage of play. The take-apart skills of the previous transitional stage make way for filling, building, stacking, and putting together. Instead of seeing objects as a "whole," children begin to notice and interact with the parts. They begin to understand shapes, sizes, and concepts that show relationships of parts. Attention span increases, and children now are ready to be introduced to crayons. When pre-writing activities are presented earlier than this stage, both you and the child will become frustrated.

Prerequisite 2 Balance

By the time children reach the constructive stage of play, usually they are sitting and standing. To begin pre-writing tasks, the child must be sitting independently. The arms must be free to interact with the crayon—not to hold up the trunk. As pre-writing skills move from random marks on the paper to the more complicated copying of shapes and letters, balance becomes an even more significant issue. The more complicated the fine motor task expected of the child, the more balance is necessary as a basis of movement. In the classroom, the child must be able to sit in an upright posture, with feet placed firmly on the floor, or on a stool or footrest. The child must be comfortable and have no fear of tipping over. Attention then will be free to focus on the task of writing.

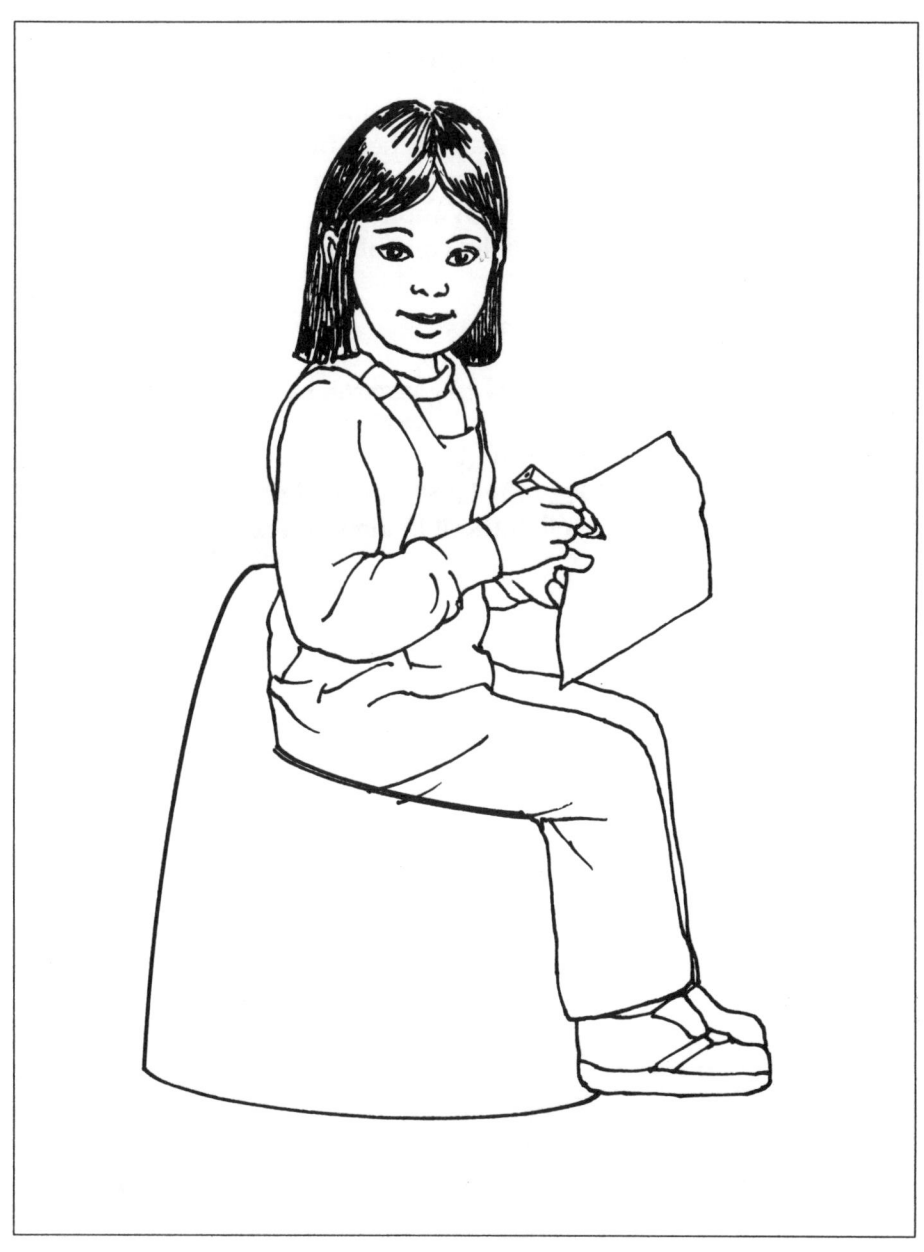

Prerequisite 3   Shoulder Stability

The ability to stabilize and control the movement of the shoulders is important for direct reaching and to provide support for the forearm, wrist, and finger actions required in holding a pencil and using it to make complex shapes. The child must be able to control the shoulders so that the arms can perform separate actions without losing precision.

Prerequisite 4   Forearm Control

The child must be able to comfortably move the forearms from a palm-down (pronated) position to a thumb-up (neutral) position. Not only must the child have the range of motion necessary to achieve these movements, but the movements must be done smoothly and with control.

Prerequisite 5   Wrist Stability

The child must be able to hold the wrists in a controlled position and to gradually move them into and out of that stable position. The wrists provide the proximal support needed for the distal or finger control used in writing. Without the easy stability provided by the wrist, the fingers have limited control.

Prerequisite 6   Grasp

The ability to grasp the hand around a writing tool is necessary for precision writing skill to develop. The ulnar (little finger) side of the hand provides the stable base from which the more active radial (thumb) side of the hand moves. The grasp needs to be firm enough to hold the pencil without being so clenched that freedom of motion is affected.

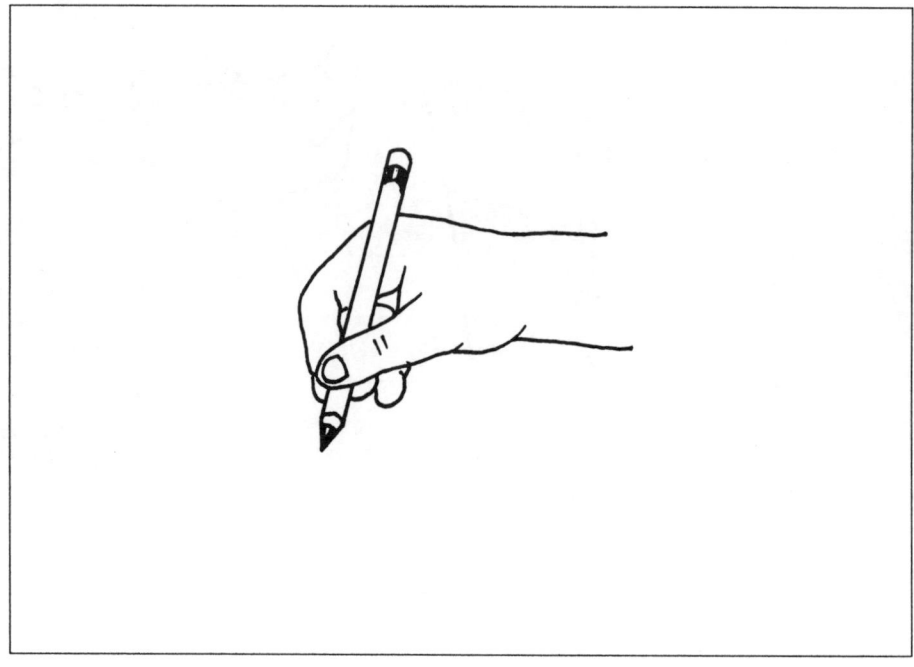

Prerequisite 7 Lead-Assist Two-Hand Usage

This is the ability to use both hands together, with one hand stabilizing while the other hand leads in the action. Children in their second year of life, who are beginning some of these pre-writing skills, have not yet established a dominant hand. When pre-writing instruction begins, interchangeable hand usage is acceptable. As children become older, they should begin to show a hand preference. Later, they will consistently hold the paper with one hand and the writing utensil with the other.

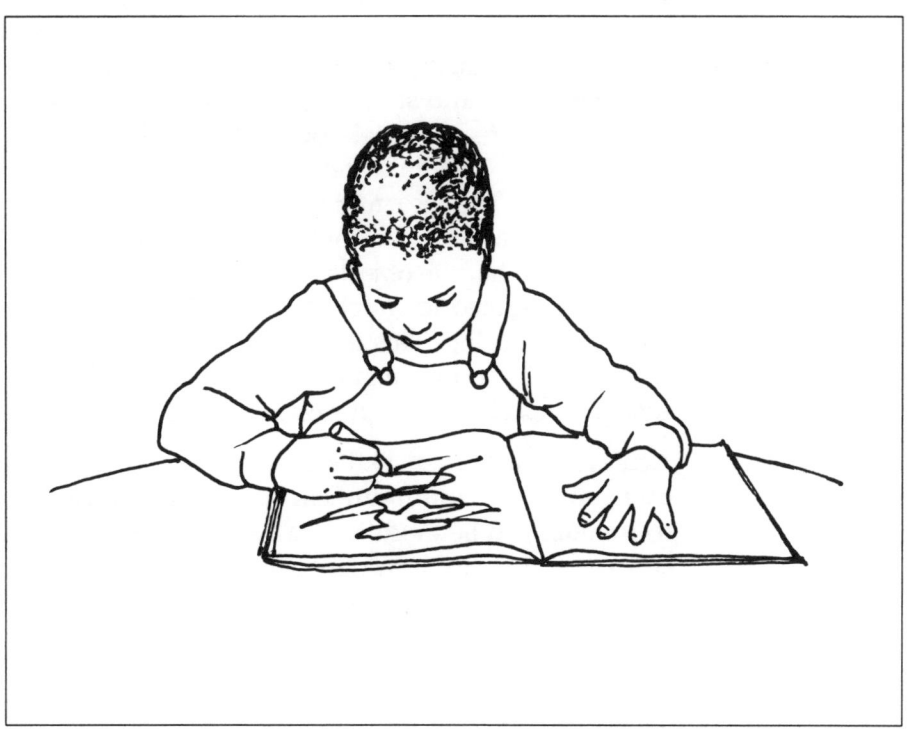

Prerequisite 8 **Coordination of Arm, Hand, and Eye Movements**

Coordinating the eyes with the finely graded actions of the shoulders, elbows, forearms, wrists, and fingers is required. Pre-writing tasks can be done without the help of vision, but they become a far more multi-sensory experience. Touch then must take over for the limited vision.

Prerequisite 9 **Sensory Experiences**

Through various sensory and motor experiences, children learn to handle a variety of materials. They refine the movement of their hands and fingers by manipulating puzzles and toys. They learn to pull toys, play with large and small objects, use both hands together, use a spoon at meals, and feel a variety of objects of different sizes, shapes, and textures. They play in water, sand, and powder, and they feel pebbles and feathers. They learn to throw accurately. All of these experiences provide preparation for holding and using a pencil. The child develops the ability to handle objects of varying size, shape, weight, and texture. The eye is trained to watch the hand movements as eye-hand coordination skills develop. This indirect preparation for writing is achieved by development and refinement of the senses of touch and sight. These sensory experiences are necessary in the child's preparation for writing.

Achievement of these skills before or while pre-writing skills are developing allows an optimum learning situation. However, instruction techniques can be modified and equipment or the environment can be adapted to help each student succeed. Methods for adapting pre-writing activities will be discussed throughout this book.

Name nine prerequisite skills for pre-writing.

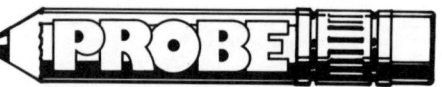

2 Developmental Stages in Acquiring Pre-Writing Skills

Children in kindergarten or first grade who are beginning to learn to write letters, numbers, and words have spent five or six years learning the pre-writing skills that prepared them for the task. The ability to master control of the pencil and to imitate and copy the lines needed for writing progresses in a sequence. Children begin with unrefined, random movements and marks, and they advance to precise imitation and control in copying specific lines in specific shapes. Preschool children learning to control a pencil or crayon usually pass through these developmental stages on their own with little notice from the adults around them. Developmentally or physically delayed children, adolescents, or adults may spend more time learning each step. To be able to succeed, they may need the help of teachers or parents in modifying the approach to the task or the writing utensils used.

Initial Stages

Stage 1 **The student mouths crayons or crinkles paper.**

These children are not yet in the constructive stage of play. They are still in the sensory explorative, or destructive, stage. They need to develop more attentive play skills before they are ready to participate in constructive pre-writing activities.

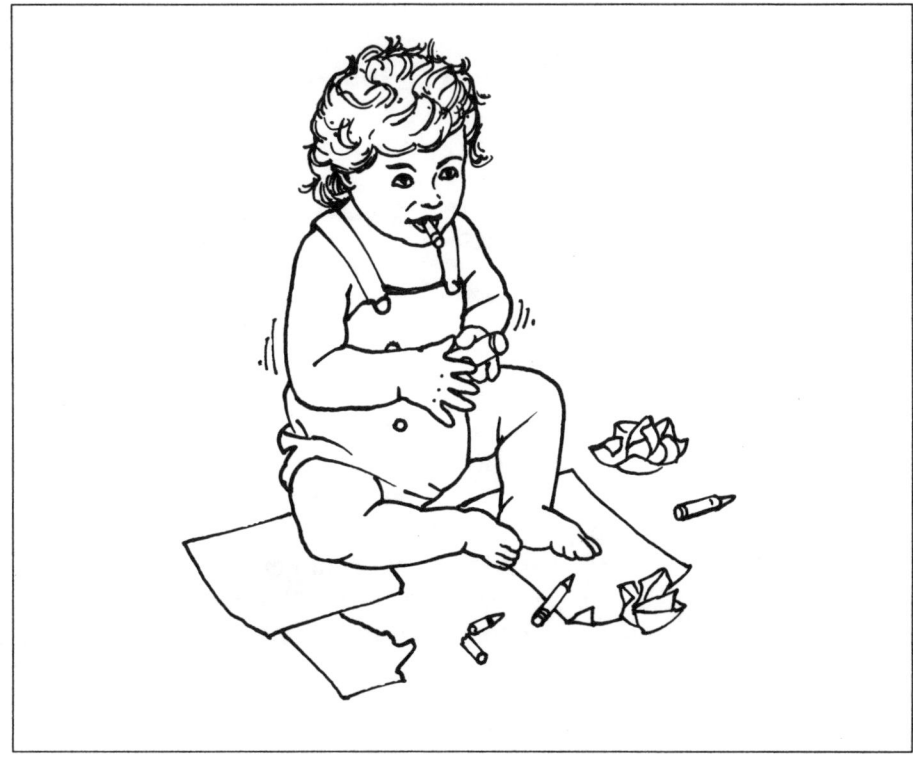

Stage 2   The student bangs crayons on paper.

These children may be ready for pre-writing activities. If banging is characteristic of all their play, they may not yet have the attention skills to try to scribble or refine their coordination. But if their other play skills are beginning to be constructive and they are building, stacking, and trying to take toys apart and put them together, this banging can be the first marks they make and can lead to random, spontaneous scribbling.

Stage 3   The student scribbles randomly.

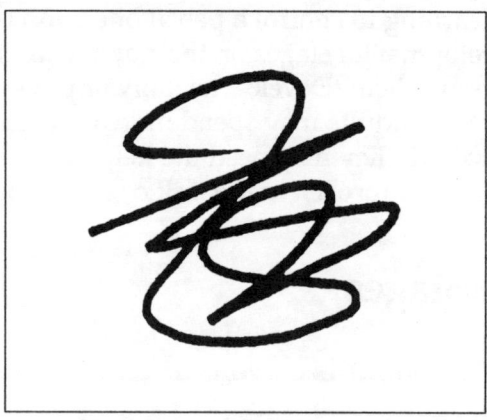

Once children have watched people write or draw with pencils or crayons and have experimented by banging crayons, they have learned that crayons are for making marks. They will pick up a crayon or pencil and begin to scribble randomly.

Stage 4a   The student scribbles spontaneously in a horizontal direction.

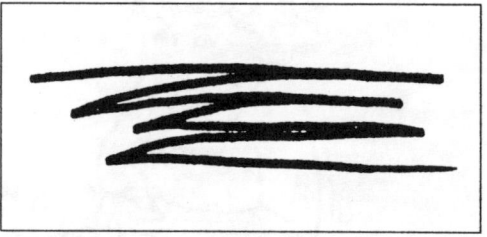

Scribbling, as a fine motor activity, serves as a task in which children further learn to control and refine their eye/hand movements. In scribbling, children perform a movement. The pencil leaves a mark on the paper that is a record of that movement. When children are encouraged to watch the movement generated by the hand and to notice the permanent record on paper of that movement, they gradually learn greater and greater control of the movement. Scribbling therefore can provide an excellent medium for improving eye/hand coordination.

Children begin to scribble in a direction, and then—as in most newly acquired play skills—they practice and practice and practice!

Children may not scribble horizontally first; their initial direction may be vertical or diagonal. Children make exceptions to every rule we create. This stage requires only a beginning *direction* to a child's scribble.

Stage 4b   **The student scribbles spontaneously in a vertical direction.**

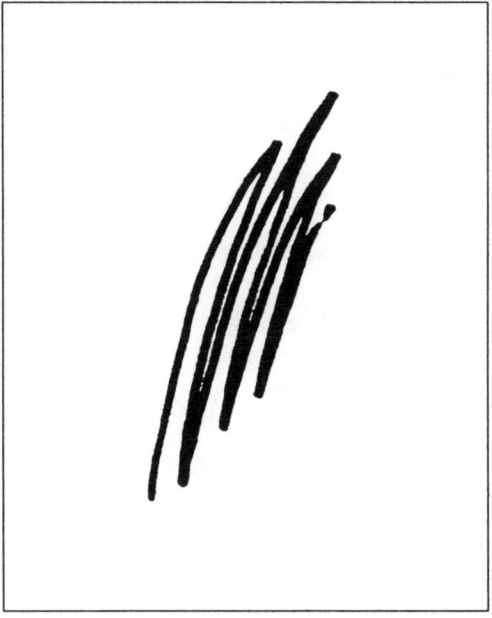

This stage may be interchanged with horizontal scribble direction as described above.

Stage 5   **The student scribbles spontaneously in a circular direction.**

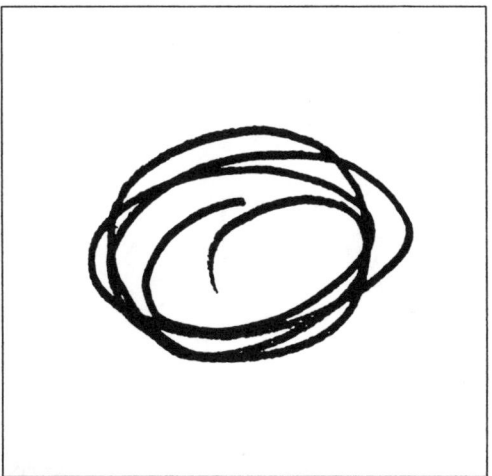

Generally, children practice circular scribbling in their play after they can repeat a horizontal or vertical scribble direction on their own. At this point, they are just practicing control and are not yet imitating.

Imitation and Copying

Once children have mastered spontaneous scribbling in horizontal, vertical, and circular directions, they are ready to begin *imitation*.

It is important here to make a distinction between imitation and copying.

In *imitation* in scribbling, the trainer makes marks while the child watches. Then the child makes marks in the same direction.

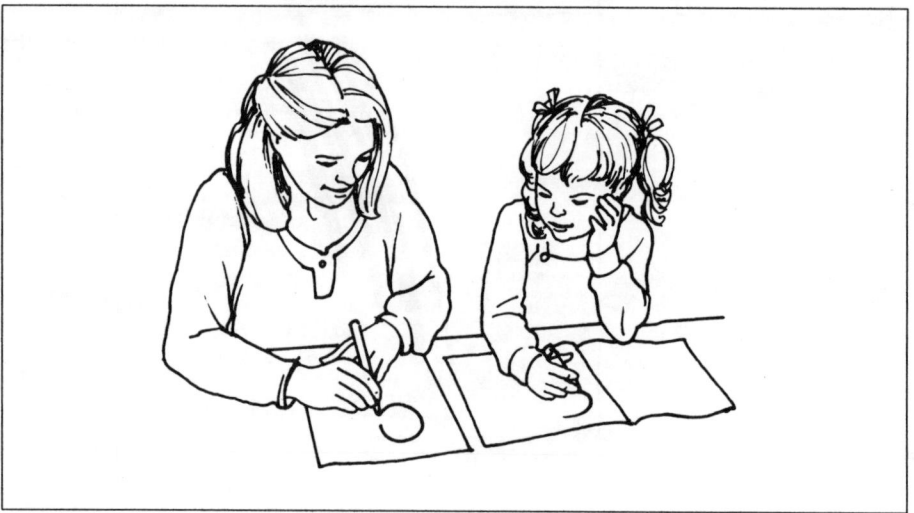

In *copying*, the trainer holds up a paper with a mark or line on it and says, "Do this" or "Make one like this." The child receives no visual cues on how to make the mark, as in imitation.

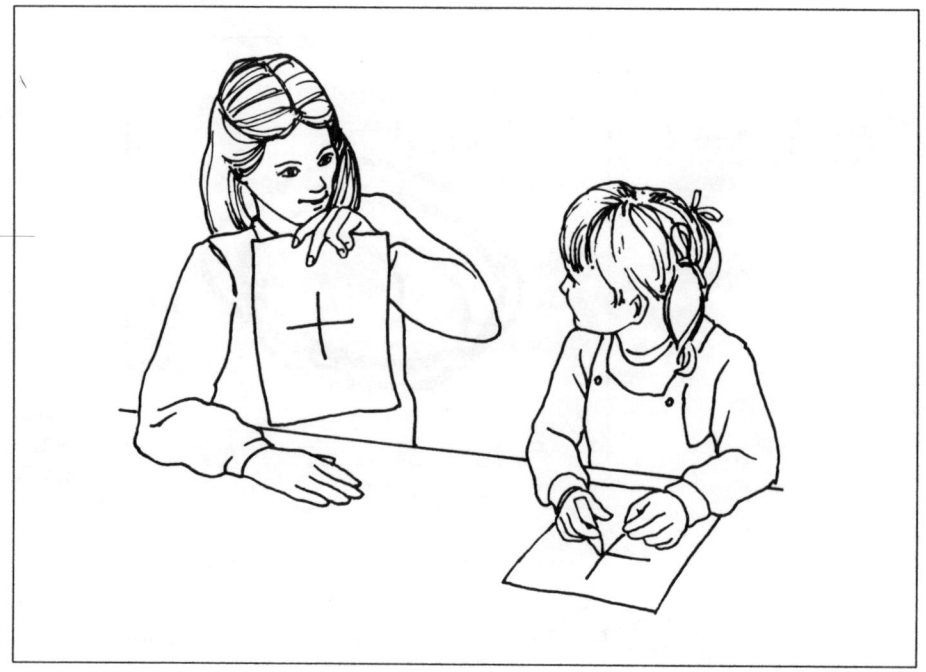

In pre-writing imitation, children are asked to imitate a movement that is already in their repertoire of movements. In other words, they are not asked to imitate a scribble direction that they have not yet demonstrated in their own scribble play.

Copying is much more difficult and should not be asked of a child who cannot imitate marks. At this stage, scribble direction and simple lines do not require much visual analysis in order to be copied. Later, as the child makes complex line combinations and shapes, the differences between imitation and copying become more pronounced.

Children imitate scribbling first. Usually the direction they *imitate* first is the direction they practiced first in their own repertoire of skills.

Stage 6a   **The student imitates a horizontal scribble direction.**

Usually the first imitated scribble direction is horizontal. Remember that this first imitation is of a scribble *direction* and not a line. Children are not yet able to make a consistent single line in scribble play; they are still in a repetitive stage of coloring.

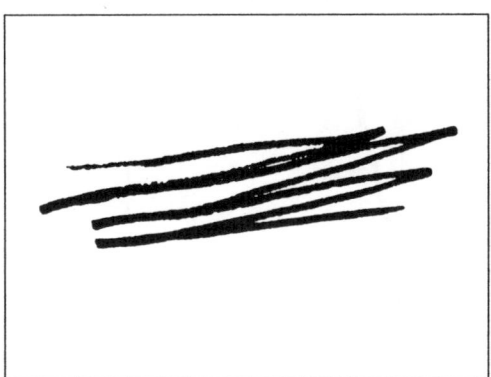

Stage 6b   **The student imitates a vertical scribble direction.**

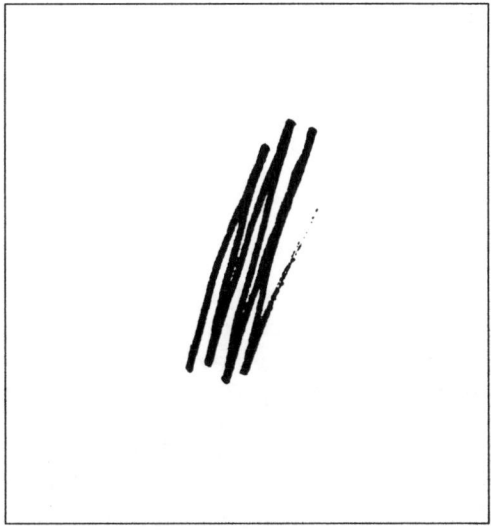

Stage 6c The student imitates a circular scribble direction.

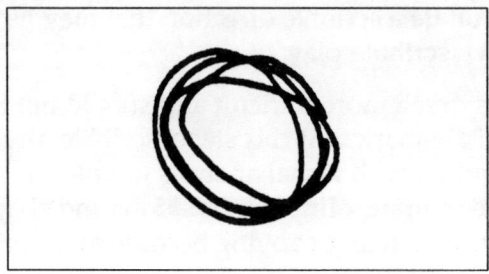

Stage 7a The student imitates a horizontal line.

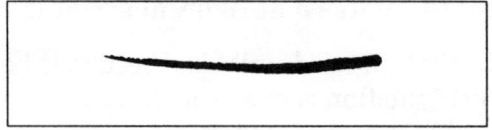

Stage 7b The student imitates a vertical line.

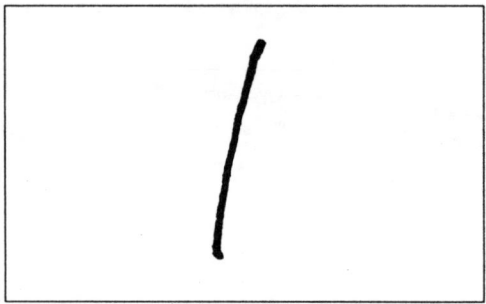

Stage 7c The student imitates a circular line.

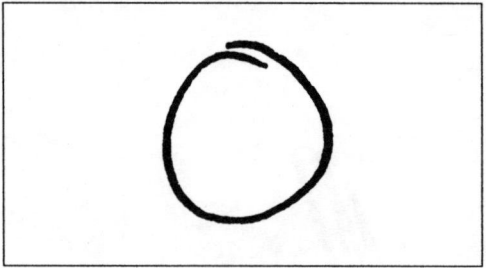

Until now, children have been imitating a direction in their scribbles but have not refined their pencil control to the point of being able to imitate a single line. In these stages they learn to imitate a single horizontal, vertical, and then circular line.

Notice that horizontal, vertical, and circular lines again are grouped together. Each child is different and will learn to imitate these lines in individualized order, depending on the child's earlier practice with scribble direction and with imitation.

Stage 8a The student copies a horizontal line.

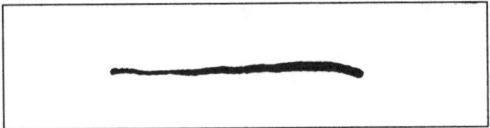

Stage 8b The student copies a vertical line.

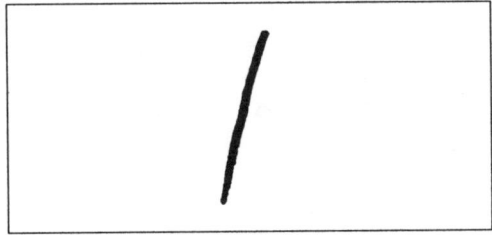

Children usually copy horizontal and vertical lines before circular lines.

Stage 9a The student copies a circle.

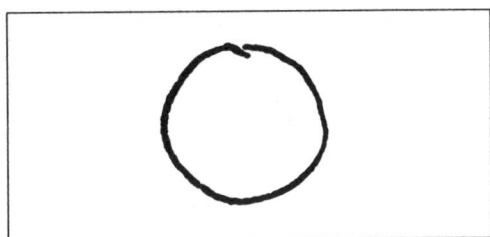

Moving from scribble direction to single lines was the first challenge in the imitation-copying sequence. Now the child must make a curved line that connects. The tendency is to continue going around and around and around! Some children have difficulty stopping their circles. This common problem will be discussed later.

Stage 9b The student imitates a cross.

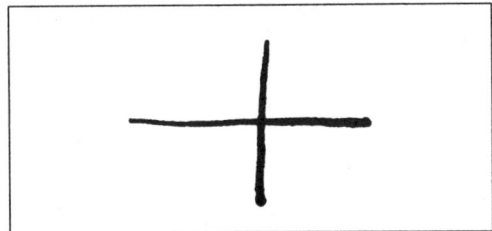

The transition from making a separate vertical and horizontal line to combining these two lines into a cross is complicated. Some children make the vertical line next to the horizontal line and don't cross them. Gradually, the lines connect into a cross.

As in most developmental sequences, children refine one skill while learning a new one. Now they can copy a circle (which they could imitate already). At the same time, they are learning to imitate a new shape, a cross.

Stage 10a   **The student copies a cross.**

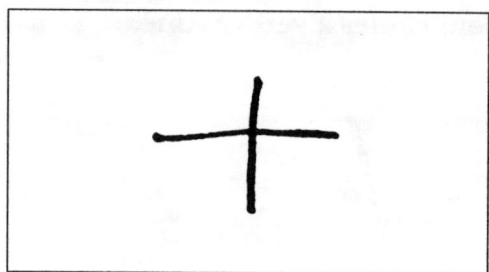

Now the child is combining two previously learned marks. The child must be able to make the visual analysis of the cross into horizontal and vertical concepts before a successful cross can be drawn.

Stage 10b   **The student imitates a right/left diagonal.**

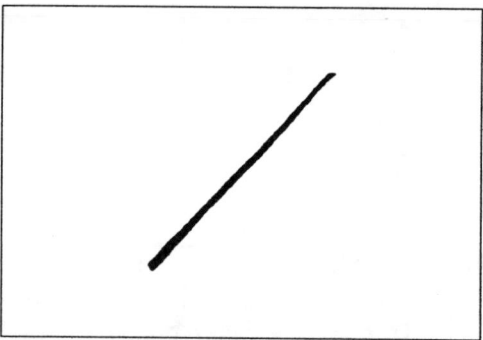

Up to this point, children have made vertical and horizontal lines. It takes more motor control and perceptual skill to make a diagonal. Children must have a more integrated awareness of their own body movements and the ability to orient themselves and the pencil in space.

Stage 11a   **The student copies a right/left diagonal.**

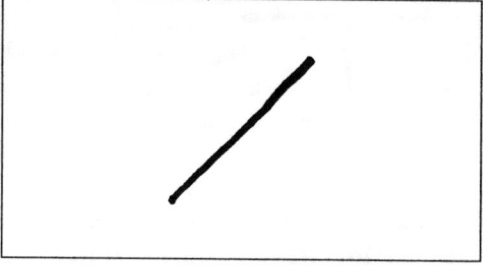

Stage 11b The student imitates a square.

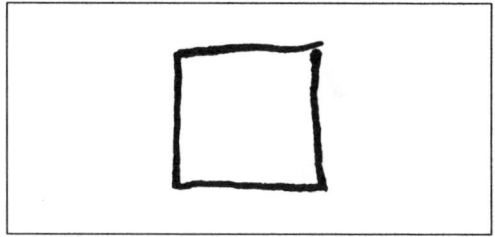

The square combines vertical and horizontal lines, which children already can make. They need to learn to visualize the lines in a square and be able to put corners together in the proper sequence to complete the shape. It is not enough perceptually just to understand the line concept here. To make closed shapes consisting of differently angled lines is a much more complex task.

Stage 12a The student copies a square.

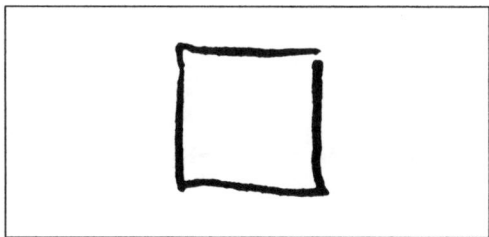

Stage 12b The student imitates a left/right diagonal.

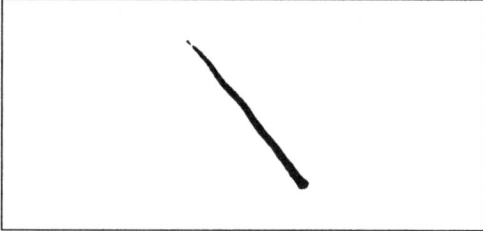

Stage 13a The student copies a left/right diagonal.

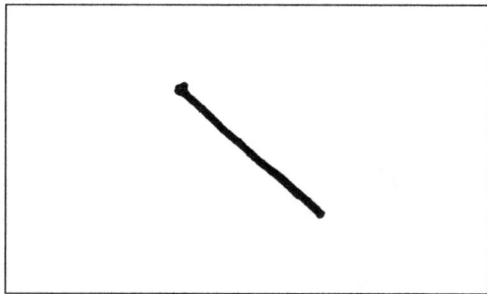

Stage 13b The student imitates an X.

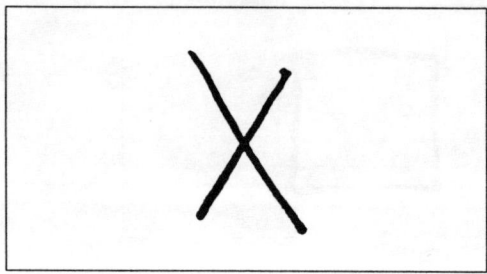

Again, the child is putting together two previously learned marks.

Stage 14a The student copies an X.

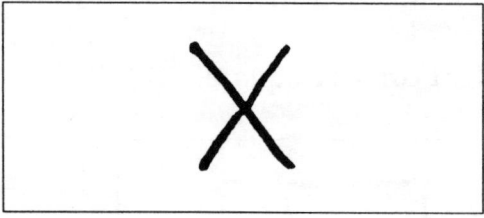

Stage 14b The student imitates a triangle.

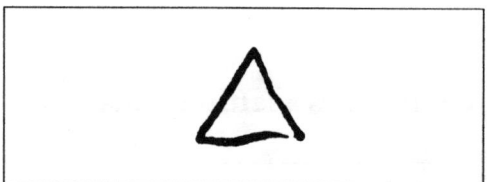

Stage 15a The student copies a triangle.

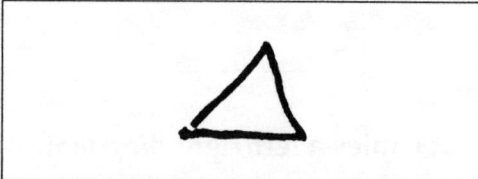

Stage 15b The student imitates a diamond.

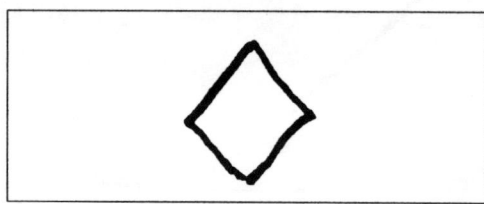

Stage 16   The student copies a diamond.

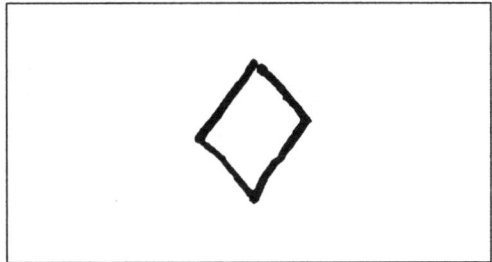

Children learn to make random marks in about the first eighteen months. They develop the motor coordination and perceptual/motor awareness to make the other imitations and copies between 3½ and 4½ years of age. After they can make the triangle and diamond, they can be expected to imitate and copy some simple letters.

This is a long developmental process, and it is hard to speed it up. Just because children can make a circle this week does not mean that they will make a cross next week, a diagonal the next, and a square the week after. They need to fully practice and experience one step and be perceptually ready before the next step comes. Teachers can expose children to the next steps, but they will go at their own rate and will not be rushed.

What is the difference between imitation and copying?

What are the developmental stages in acquiring pre-writing skills?

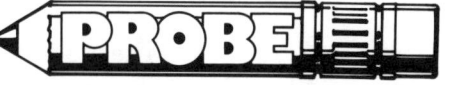

Overview of Pre-Writing Developmental Stages

Stage 1	The student mouths crayons or crinkles paper.
Stage 2	The student bangs crayons on paper.
Stage 3	The student scribbles randomly.
Stage 4a	The student scribbles spontaneously in a horizontal direction.
Stage 4b	The student scribbles spontaneously in a vertical direction.
Stage 5	The student scribbles spontaneously in a circular direction.
Stage 6a	The student imitates a horizontal scribble direction.
Stage 6b	The student imitates a vertical scribble direction.
Stage 6c	The student imitates a circular scribble direction.
Stage 7a	The student imitates a horizontal line.
Stage 7b	The student imitates a vertical line.
Stage 7c	The student imitates a circular line.
Stage 8a	The student copies a horizontal line.
Stage 8b	The student copies a vertical line.
Stage 9a	The student copies a circle.
Stage 9b	The student imitates a cross.
Stage 10a	The student copies a cross.
Stage 10b	The student imitates a right/left diagonal.
Stage 11a	The student copies a right/left diagonal.
Stage 11b	The student imitates a square.
Stage 12a	The student copies a square.
Stage 12b	The student imitates a left/right diagonal.
Stage 13a	The student copies a left/right diagonal.
Stage 13b	The student imitates an X.
Stage 14a	The student copies an X.
Stage 14b	The student imitates a triangle.
Stage 15a	The student copies a triangle.
Stage 15b	The student imitates a diamond.
Stage 16	The student copies a diamond.

Checklist for Assessing Pre-Writing Developmental Skills

Student's Name _____

Date of Assessment		Developmental Stage	Date Achieved
	1	The student mouths crayons or crinkles paper.	
	2	The student bangs crayons on paper.	
	3	The student scribbles randomly.	
	4a	The student scribbles spontaneously in a horizontal direction.	
	4b	The student scribbles spontaneously in a vertical direction.	
	5	The student scribbles spontaneously in a circular direction.	
	6a	The student *imitates* a horizontal scribble direction.	
	6b	The student *imitates* a vertical scribble direction.	
	6c	The student *imitates* a circular scribble direction.	
	7a	The student *imitates* a horizontal line.	
	7b	The student *imitates* a vertical line.	
	7c	The student *imitates* a circular line.	
	8a	The student *copies* a horizontal line.	
	8b	The student *copies* a vertical line.	
	9a	The student *copies* a circle.	
	9b	The student *imitates* a cross.	
	10a	The student *copies* a cross.	
	10b	The student *imitates* a right/left diagonal.	
	11a	The student *copies* a right/left diagonal.	
	11b	The student *imitates* a square.	
	12a	The student *copies* a square.	
	12b	The student *imitates* a left/right diagonal.	

© 1990 by Communication Skill Builders, Inc.
This page may be reproduced for administrative use.

Date of Assessment		Developmental Stage	Date Achieved
	13a	The student *copies* a left/right diagonal.	
	13b	The student *imitates* an X.	
	14a	The student *copies* an X.	
	14b	The student *imitates* a triangle.	
	15a	The student *copies* a triangle.	
	15b	The student *imitates* a diamond.	
	16	The student *copies* a diamond.	

Date _____

Comments _____

_____

_____

_____

_____

_____

_____

_____

_____

_____

_____

_____

_____

_____

_____

_____

© 1990 by Communication Skill Builders, Inc.
This page may be reproduced for administrative use.

3 Developmental Stages in Learning to Color

The development and refinement of pre-writing skills, including pencil control and the ability to imitate and copy strokes and lines, directly relate to children's interest in coloring pictures and their ability to do so. Similarly, the refinement and control that children learn in coloring strokes and staying within defined areas reinforce the pre-writing skills they are simultaneously learning.

Once children can imitate and copy vertical, horizontal, and circular strokes, they may begin to show an interest in coloring pictures. Children follow a general developmental sequence in learning to color *picture areas*, as they do with pre-writing strokes.

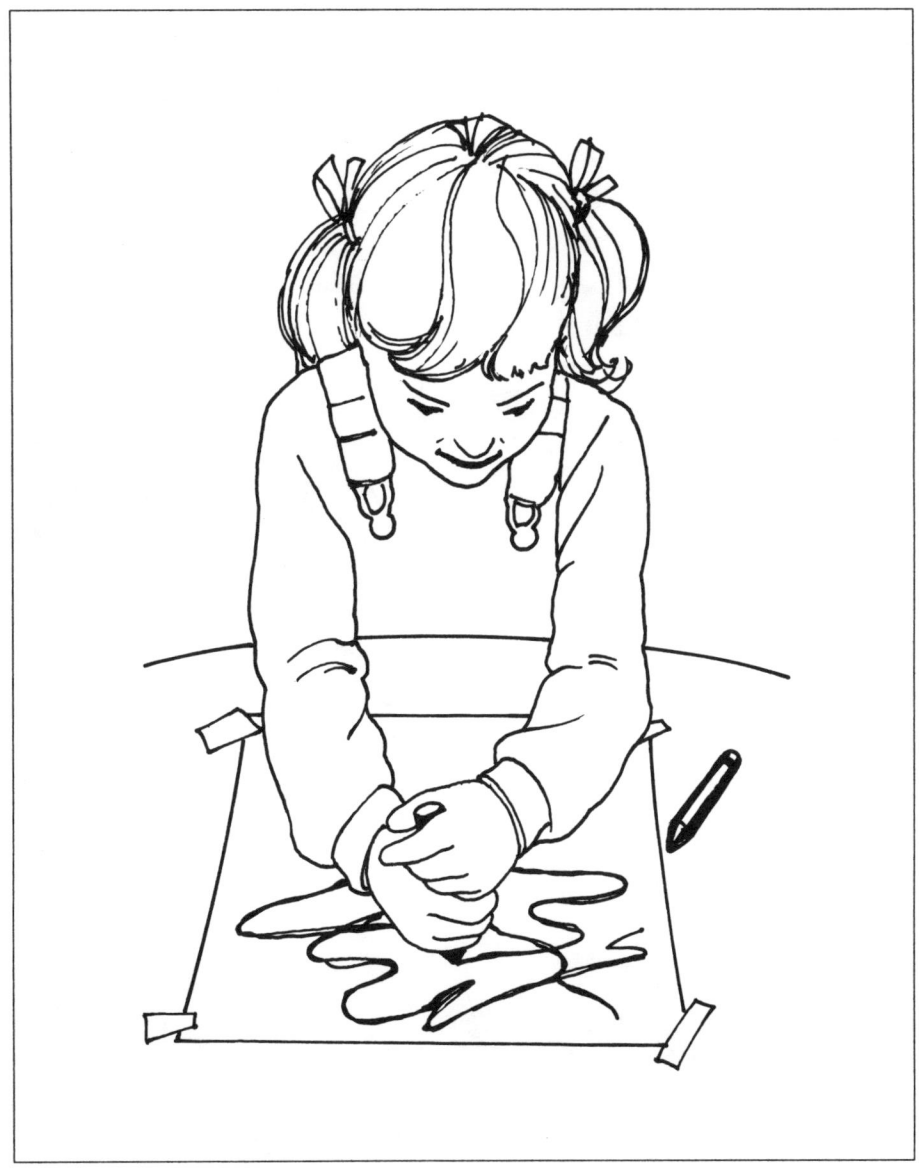

Picture Area

Stage 1 **The student covers a large paper with color.**

At this first stage, children make crayon contact with a large piece of paper. They know that they want to color the page, yet they are just as likely to color the table, wall, or floor around the paper as they are to color the paper itself.

Stage 2 **The student covers an 8½" x 11" piece of paper with color.**

At this stage, children have gained increased control of the shoulder, arm, and hand. They have simultaneously begun to understand that the paper, not the table, is for coloring. Perhaps mother (or teacher) has helped to reinforce this notion.

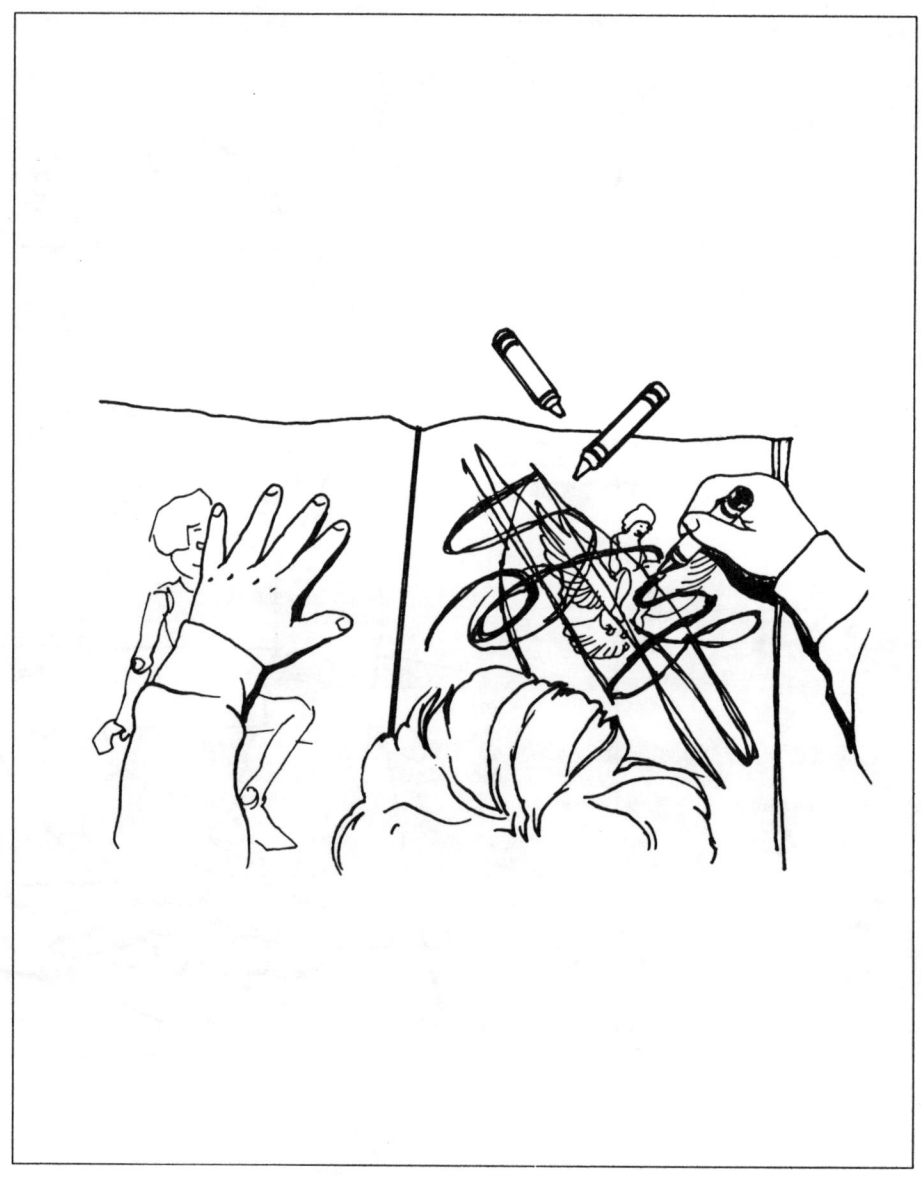

Stage 3 **The student colors a medium-sized area or picture (a 6-inch circle, square, or other simple geometric shape).**

Children are now increasing their arm and hand control, their ability to color with strokes, and their understanding that lined pictures are for coloring. They will stay relatively within the outer lines of the drawing, but with no discrimination yet for inside detail. If a 6-inch geometric shape is presented, they will stay approximately within the area. If a picture of that size is presented, such as a drawing of a house or a child playing, children will color without trying to stay within the design but will stay within the 6-inch area.

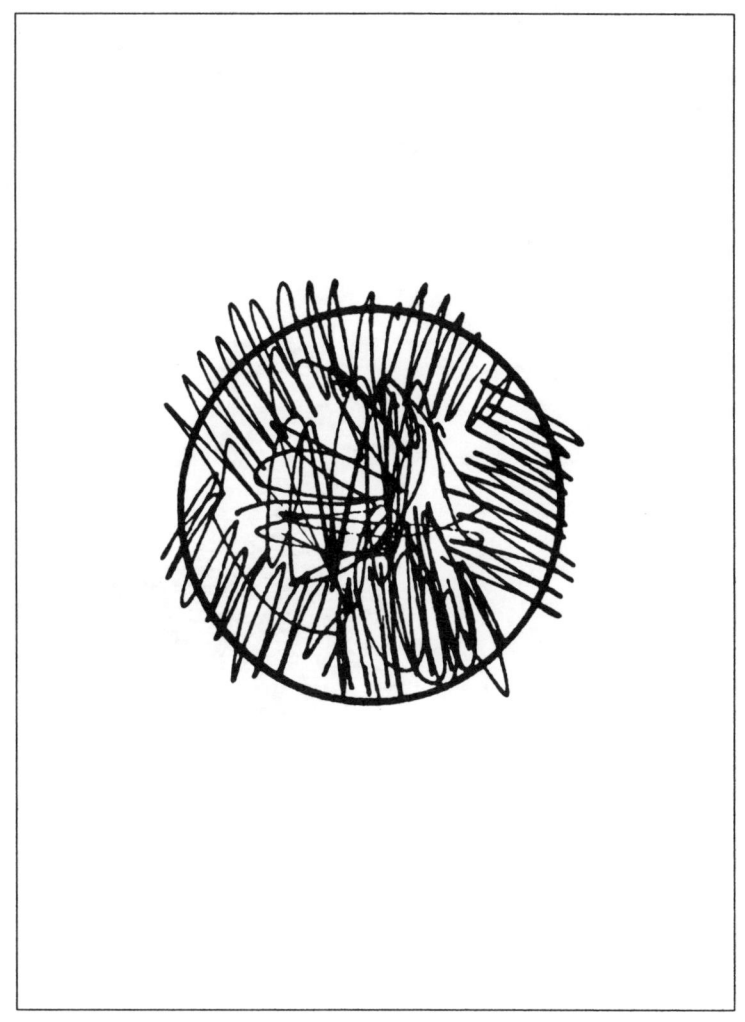

Stage 4 **The student colors a small area (a 2-inch circle or other simple geometric shape).**

Children now can color a smaller area, staying within the outside limits. Coordination and motor control have increased. Inside detail is not yet precise.

Stage 5 **The student colors a medium-sized design.**

This stage seems to occur almost simultaneously with the previous stage. A 5- to 8-inch picture can be colored without straying beyond the confines of the outside line.

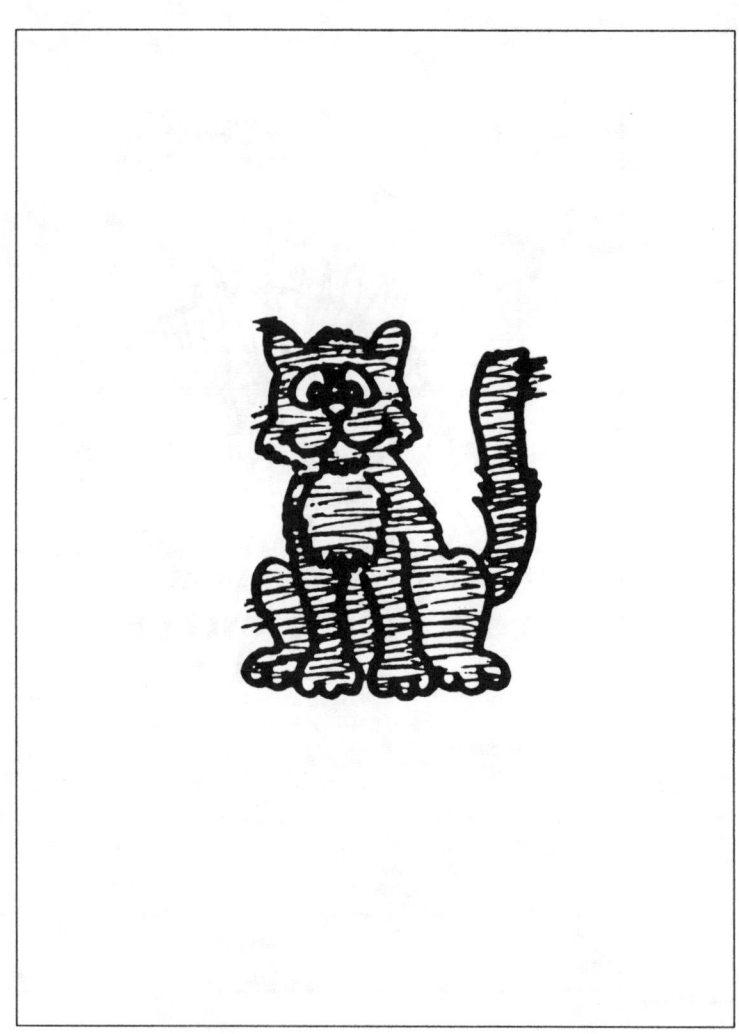

Stage 6 **The student colors a small design with accurate attention to detail.**

Now children can color any picture presented, staying within the lines and making appropriate stroke and color adjustments to details.

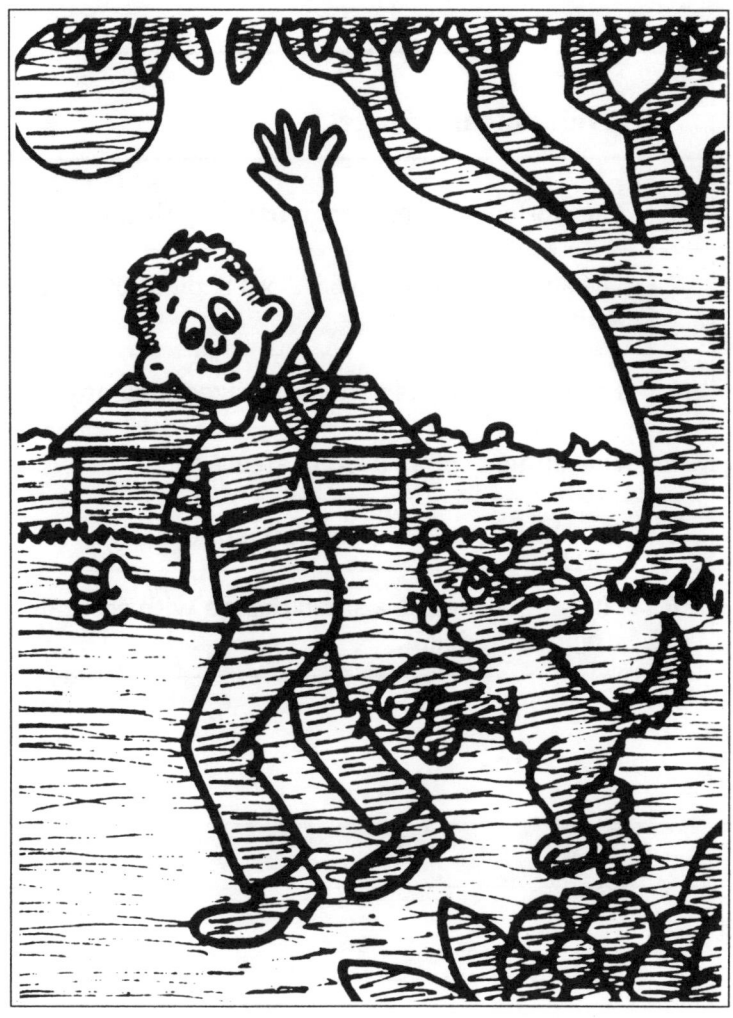

What are the six stages in learning
to color a picture area?

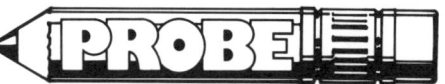

Checklist for Assessing Ability to Color a Picture Area

Student's Name_____

Date of Assessment		Developmental Stage	Date Achieved
	1	The student covers a large paper with color.	
	2	The student covers an 8½" x 11" piece of paper with color.	
	3	The student colors a medium-sized area or picture.	
	4	The student colors a small area.	
	5	The student colors a medium-sized design.	
	6	The student colors a small design with accurate attention to detail.	

Date_____

Comments_____

_____
_____
_____
_____
_____
_____
_____
_____
_____
_____
_____

© 1990 Communication Skill Builders, Inc.
This page may be reproduced for administrative use.

Stroke Control

While children are refining their motor abilities and eye/hand coordination to color within a smaller and smaller picture area, they also are refining their stroke control. Development of stroke control follows an observable sequence.

Stage 1 **The student colors with random lines.**

Initially, children have no stroke control. Their pencil grasp probably is immature and their stroke lines are random. No attention is given yet to coloring within any confines of a picture—or even a paper.

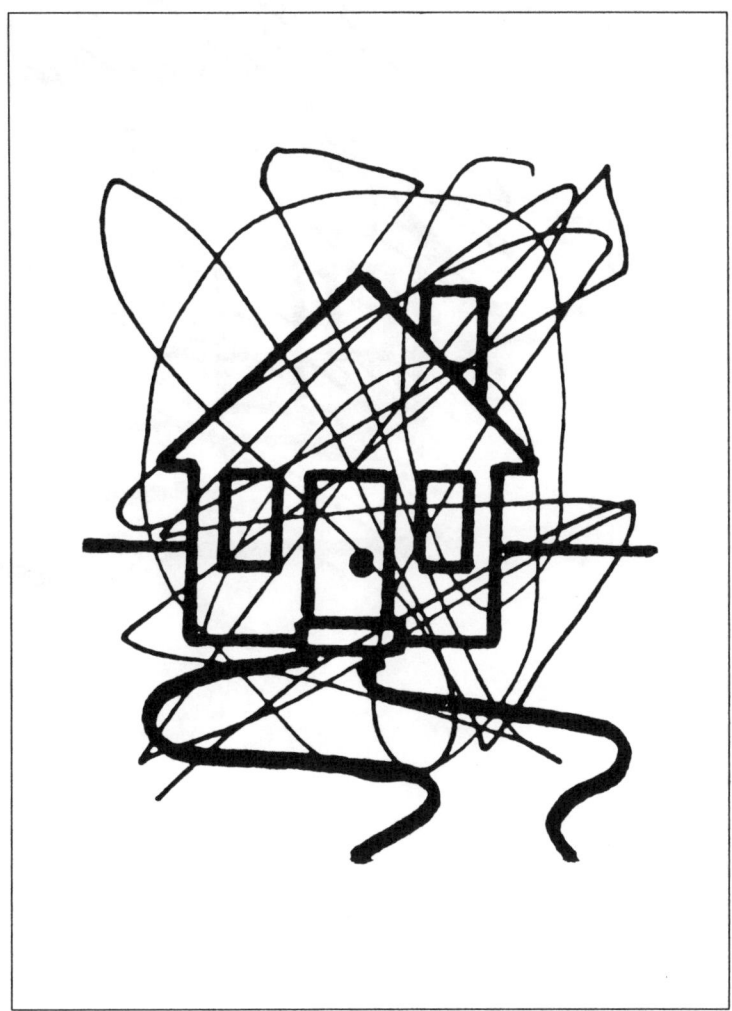

Stage 2 **The student colors grossly within a medium-sized picture, using one stroke direction.**

About the time that children are gaining the eye/hand coordination necessary to stay within a medium-sized picture, they also are gaining stroke control. They will stay within the lines, stroking in only one direction.

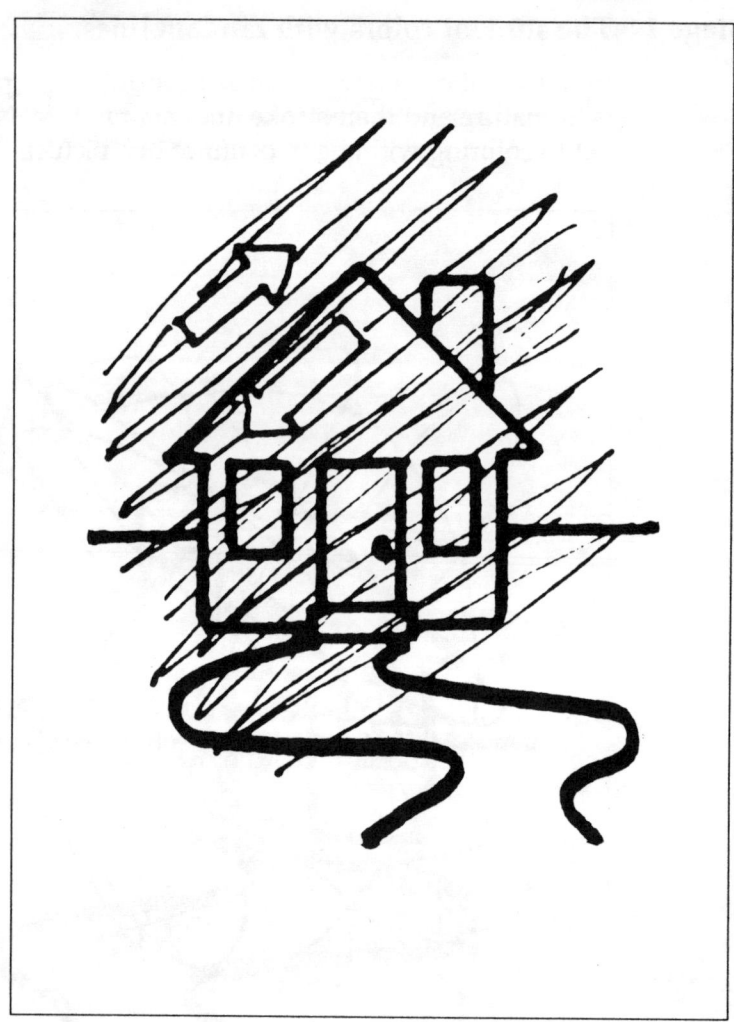

Stage 3   The student accommodates the paper to fit the stroke direction.

Children watch others coloring, and they try to imitate staying within the designated picture lines. They have only one stroke direction that they can control. So instead of turning the wrist in a coordinated fashion to change their stroke to match the picture shape, they use the one stroke and turn the paper where appropriate to make a different stroke.

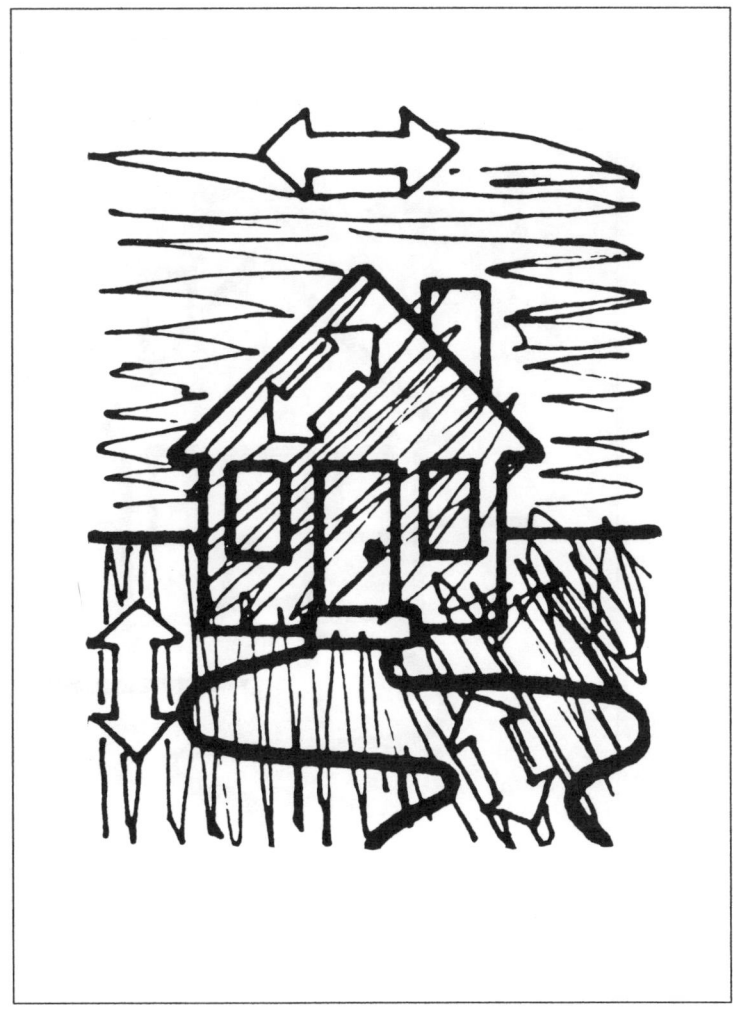

Stage 4 **The student adjusts the stroke to fit the area, keeping the paper still.**

Children begin to be able to keep the paper still and change their own stroke by moving the fingers and wrist in appropriate combinations. It is interesting to watch the contortions children get into during this stage as they refine the coordinated combinations of movements needed by shoulders, elbows, wrists, and fingers.

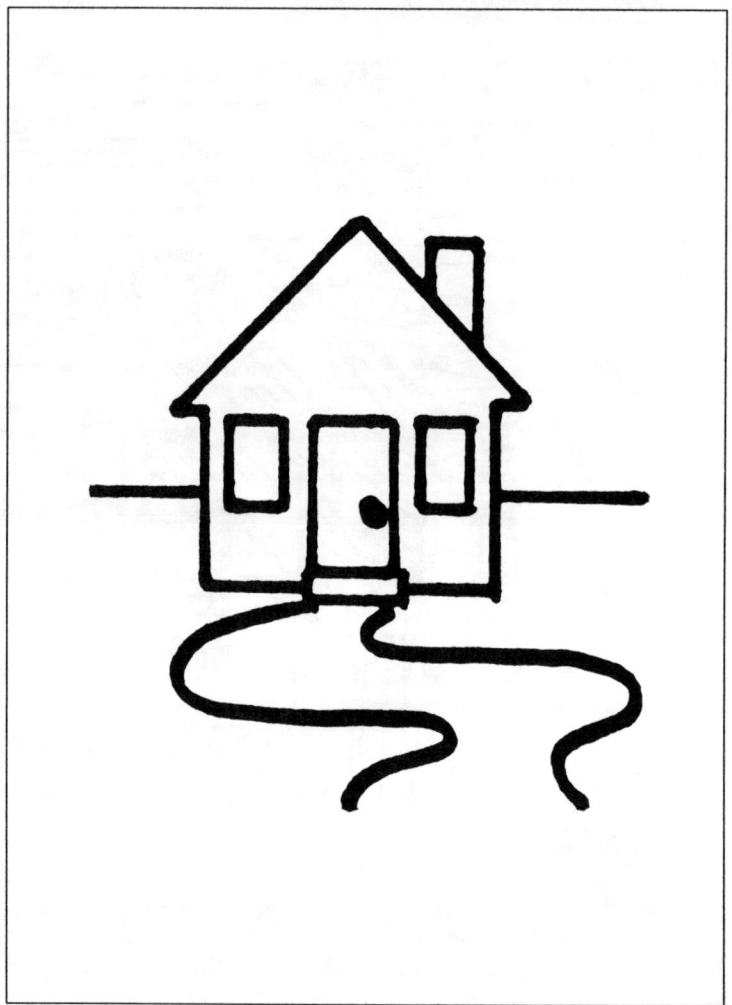

What are the four stages in learning stroke control in coloring?

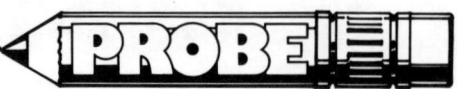

Checklist for Assessing Ability to Control Stroke

Student's Name _____

Date of Assessment		Developmental Stage	Date Achieved
	1	The student colors with random lines.	
	2	The student colors grossly within a medium-sized picture, using one stroke direction.	
	3	The student accommodates the paper to fit the stroke direction.	
	4	The student adjusts the stroke to fit the area, keeping the paper still.	

Date _____

Comments _____

_____
_____
_____
_____
_____
_____
_____
_____
_____
_____
_____
_____

Use of Color

As children gain motor coordination and perceptual/motor control of the crayon or writing utensil, they increase their awareness of the appropriateness of color usage. Learning to use color follows an observable developmental pattern.

Stage 1 **The student uses color randomly, with one color per picture.**

At this stage, when children color all over an 8 1/2" x 11" piece of paper (and onto the table) with random strokes, generally they use a random crayon color. They are just as likely to choose an orange crayon to color a picture of a boy riding a bicycle as they are to choose a brown one. As they begin to develop a direction to their stroke, they still have no regard for color appropriateness.

Stage 2 **The student uses color randomly, with several colors per picture.**

As children become able to control their directional stroke to stay within a medium-sized picture, often they begin to introduce a second or third color. The picture may end up with gross strokes, several colors, and still no appropriateness of color. (The tree may have purple, orange, and red sections.)

Stage 3 **The student begins to use some colors appropriately.**

Children now can stay within the outer lines of a medium-sized picture. They can change colors and begin to select some appropriate ones. (The girl's hair may be red instead of green, but the eyes may be yellow or pink.)

Stage 4 **The student uses color appropriately.**

Children now can color small areas with attention to detail. They accommodate their movements to make appropriate strokes. Colors are used appropriately.

What are the four developmental stages in learning to use color?

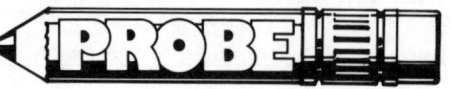

Checklist for Assessing Ability to Use Color

Student's Name _____

Date of Assessment		Developmental Stage	Date Achieved
	1	The student uses color randomly, with one color per picture.	
	2	The student uses color randomly, with several colors per picture.	
	3	The student begins to use some colors appropriately.	
	4	The student uses color appropriately.	

Date _____

Comments _____

_____

_____

_____

_____

_____

_____

_____

_____

_____

_____

_____

_____

© 1990 Communication Skill Builders, Inc.
This page may be reproduced for administrative use.

Overview of Coloring Skills Development

This chart shows a total picture of the relationship between the three coloring skills.

Picture Area	Stroke Control	Use of Color
Covers large paper with color	Uses random lines	
Covers an 8 1/2" x 11" paper with color	Colors grossly, using one stroke direction	Uses random color
Colors medium-sized area (geometric)	Colors with more consistent direction	Uses several colors
Colors small area (geometric)	Accommodates paper to stroke	Begins to use some appropriate colors
Colors medium-sized design		
Colors small design with attention to detail	Adjusts stroke, keeping paper still	Uses appropriate colors

4 Choosing Appropriate Pre-Writing Materials

Pre-writing activities do not have to be taught at a table, using a crayon or pencil and paper. Materials can be used that stimulate visual, tactile, olfactory, auditory, proprioceptive, vestibular, and even taste sensations. A varied approach can increase the child's interest level. Try changing the pre-writing tool and surface daily to give the child continually new sensory experiences.

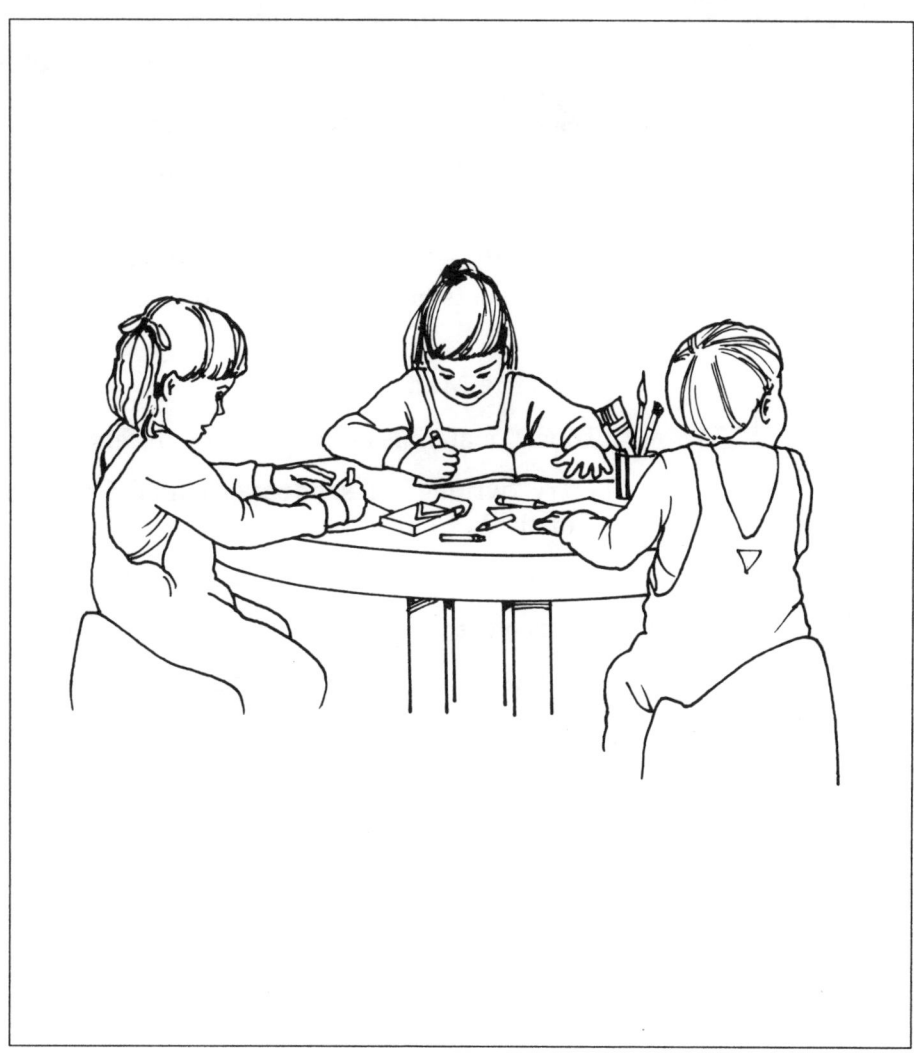

Sensory Media

Various sensory media can be used in pre-writing activities in many different combinations. Use your imagination, and neither you nor your students will get bored.

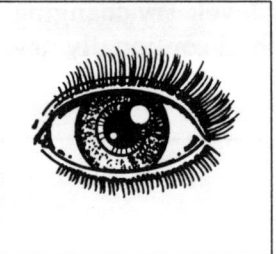

■ Visual Media

— Try "writing" on:
  Aluminum foil.
  Construction paper of different colors.
  Different kinds of paper (brown paper bags, butcher paper, waxed paper).
  Standard paper or coloring books.

— Use special coloring books in which the color appears when children paint with water.

— Use different colors of chalk, markers, crayons, pens, pencils, and paints (including finger paints, watercolors, or tempera).

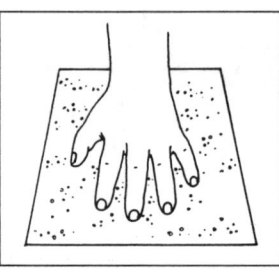

■ Tactile Media

"Touch" materials can have many different textures and temperatures.

— Try "writing" on sandpaper with different crayons, paintbrushes, or chalk.

— Draw around sandpaper or wooden stencils.

— Trace with a finger around a shape made of yarn or a craft stick.

— Try drawing in sand or mud.

— Use lotions, pudding, gelatin, oatmeal, or whipped cream to finger paint.

— Change the temperature of the materials. Sometimes put the paint or markers or crayons in the refrigerator before the activity. Lotion can be warmed in a microwave oven.

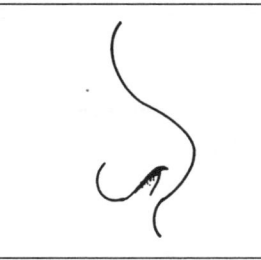

■ Olfactory Media

The sense of smell can be incorporated into pre-writing tasks.

— Try drawing with scented markers.

— Add a few drops of bubble bath or scented oil to homemade finger paint. (See the recipes on page 44.)

— Add vanilla, mint, or cherry flavoring to finger paints—but be careful! The smell is so good that children may want to taste the paint. Use it on edible finger paint only.

— Use scented lotions for finger painting.

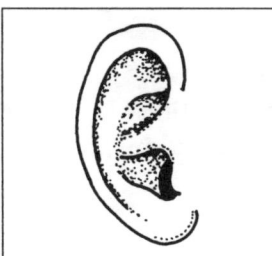

■ Auditory Media

Pre-writing activities can even include an auditory component.

— Use a musical toothbrush to paint.

— Attach bells to the end of a paintbrush.

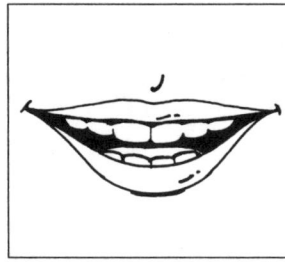

■ Gustatory Media

Even the sense of taste can be incorporated in pre-writing activities for young children.

— Try finger painting in whipping cream on a flat pan of gelatin.

— Try drawing on a frosted cake to decorate it.

— Draw with cheese spread on crackers or bread.

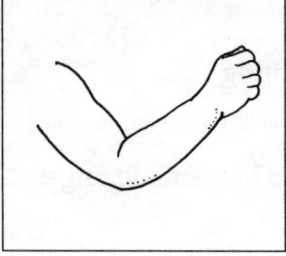

Proprioceptive Media

Proprioceptive media are those that stimulate joint muscle feedback. They include activities in which there is increased weight or resistance or two-hand involvement with the pre-writing tool.

— Use a weighted paintbrush.

— Use a paper-towel roll as a wand, and draw in the air with both hands.

— Use a scarf to make lines or circles in the air.

Vestibular Media

Activities in which the child has to move and change position also affect the vestibular, or balancing, system. These will be described in Chapter 7, Movement and Pre-Writing Skills.

Name several ways to vary pre-writing activities to include:

— Visual stimulation
— Tactile stimulation
— Olfactory stimulation
— Auditory stimulation
— Gustatory stimulation
— Proprioceptive stimulation

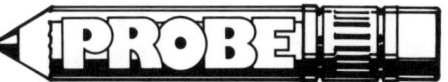

Recipes for Finger Paint

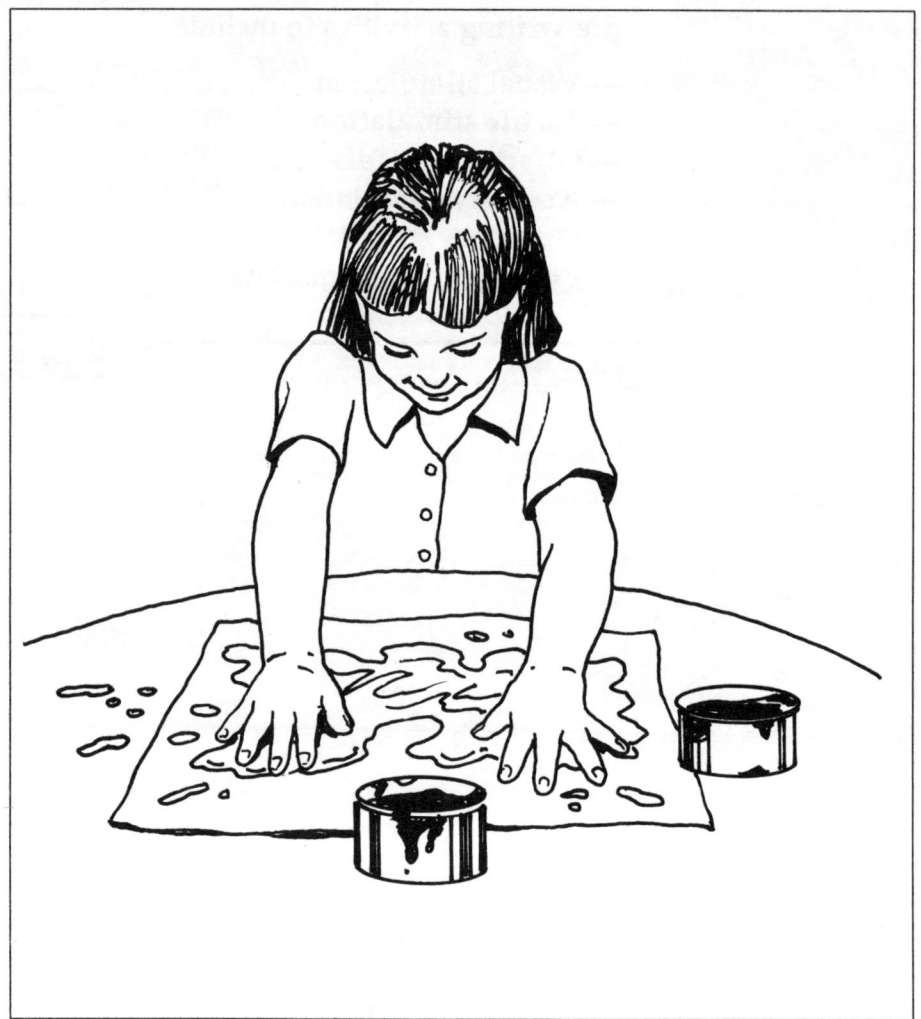

■ Ivory Snow Flakes Finger Paint

Combine Ivory Snow Flakes with enough water to make the mixture "gloppy." Mix with whisk or electric beater until it is gooey finger-paint texture. (Optional: Add food coloring.)

■ Cornstarch Finger Paint

Put 2 cups of cornstarch in a pan and add water, while stirring, until it is of glue consistency. Cook this mixture, stirring constantly, to a clear gel consistency. Cool. (Optional: Add food coloring or flavoring.) This is a great texture!

■ Flour/Salt Finger Paint

Combine 1 cup flour, 4 teaspoons salt, and $7/8$ cup cold water. Add food coloring or tempera paint. Mix well. Store in refrigerator.

5 Adaptive Techniques for Problem Areas

We have examined the normal developmental sequences of learning pre-writing skills, learning to color, and making strokes. Most children breeze through these stages with little assistance; but some children may need help if they are to succeed at pre-writing activities. You may encounter many common problems as you try to help your students move through the developmental stages of pre-writing.

All pieces of equipment mentioned in this section will be described in more detail later.

Problem Area: Balance

For some children, balance may be a problem. They may have an immaturely developed motor system, or they may have a diagnosed disability such as cerebral palsy, apraxia, or other type of learning disorder. It can be very difficult for these children to concentrate on the refined perceptual motor tasks if they are seated poorly. When balance is stressed, a child's attention moves to the feeling of falling over rather than to the writing activity you are presenting.

There are several factors to consider when choosing the position in which a child participates in a pre-writing task. In general, a rule of thumb is to position the child in the most stable, comfortable position possible when teaching a new or complicated perceptual motor task. Let the child play with a variety of different positions when practicing an already learned or simpler skill.

■ Stable Seating Options

To be positioned in a stable or well-supported fashion, several positions may be considered.

Prone or Tummy Lying

In this position, the child's whole body, elbows, forearms, and wrists are supported. The child does not need to fear falling over or tipping out of the chair. The position provides an excellent base of support from which to perform new, challenging fine motor tasks.

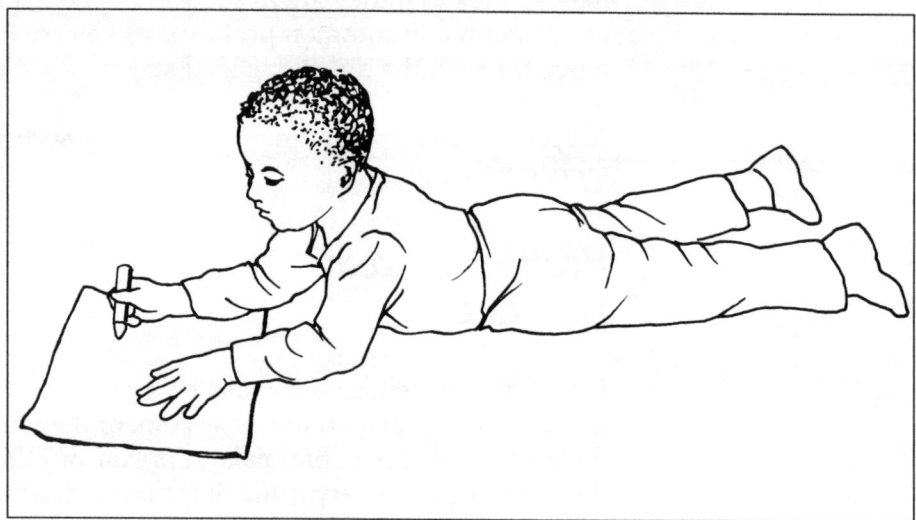

Chair Sitting

When using school desks and tables, be sure the child is seated with feet firmly on the floor or on a footrest or short stool. Dangling feet—a common problem in schools—provide poor support for sitting. Some children who have more severe balance problems may need to sit in an armchair with extra cushions at their sides.

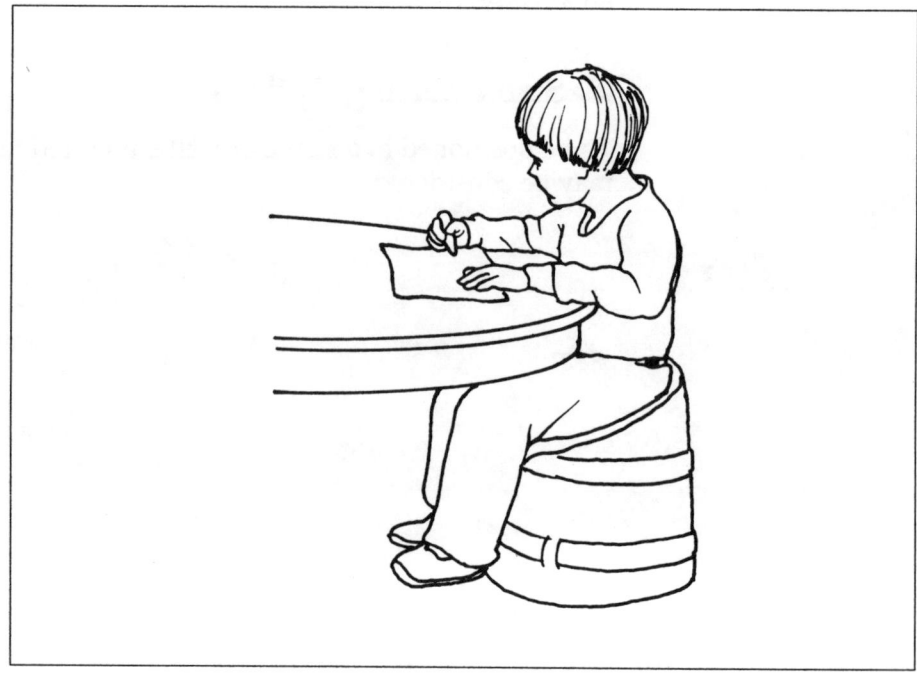

■ **Practice Seating Options**

Practice seating options are those that challenge the child's balance slightly. These positions depend on the skills of the individual child and should be used only when practicing already learned skills or skills that require less concentration or precision.

Standing

This can be an excellent change from the usual table-and-chair position in the classroom. Use it at the chalkboard or an easel or when doing a group project on butcher paper taped to the wall. This position can provide opportunities to reach forward and up and thereby stretch muscles that otherwise would be resting on the table.

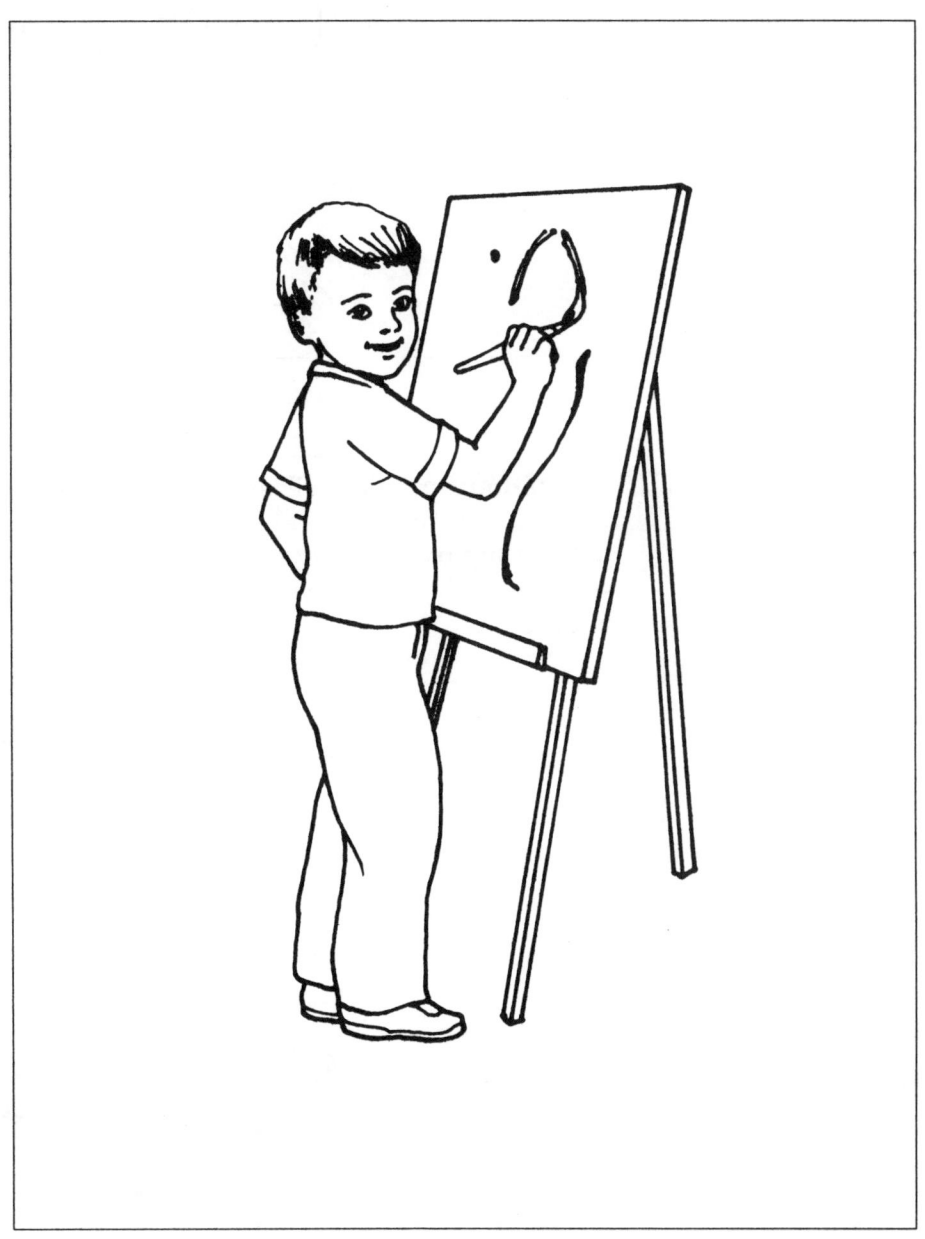

Kneeling

The child can kneel at a table or low easel. Some teachers bring towels to fold as knee pads. This position has the advantage of straightening the hips.

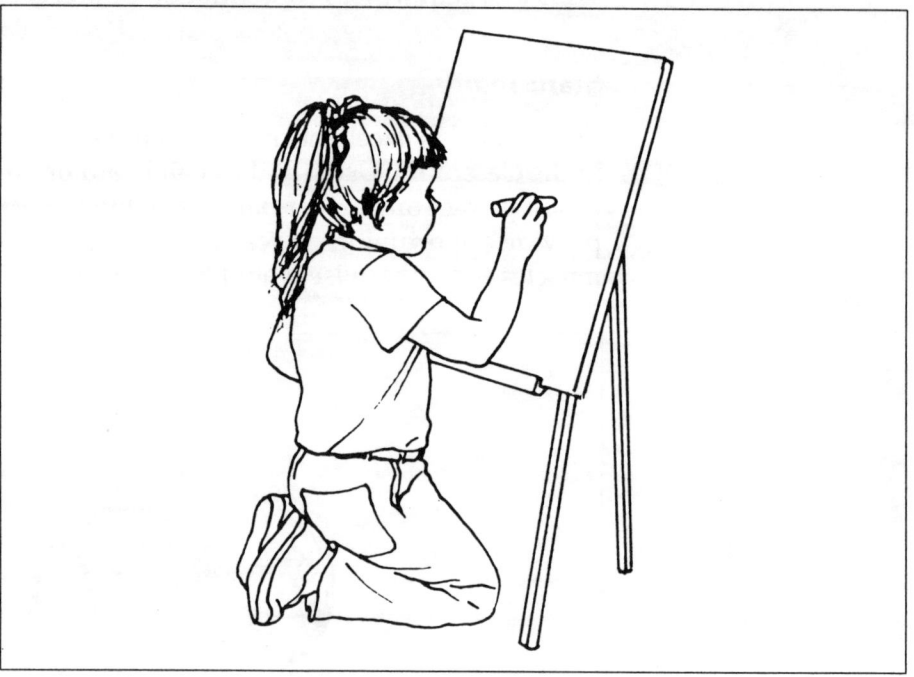

Quadraped

This all-fours position will seem like something new for children who are used to sitting at tables. It is an excellent position for doing classroom group projects. Several children in this position around a large sheet of butcher paper will have plenty of room to draw or color a part of the picture.

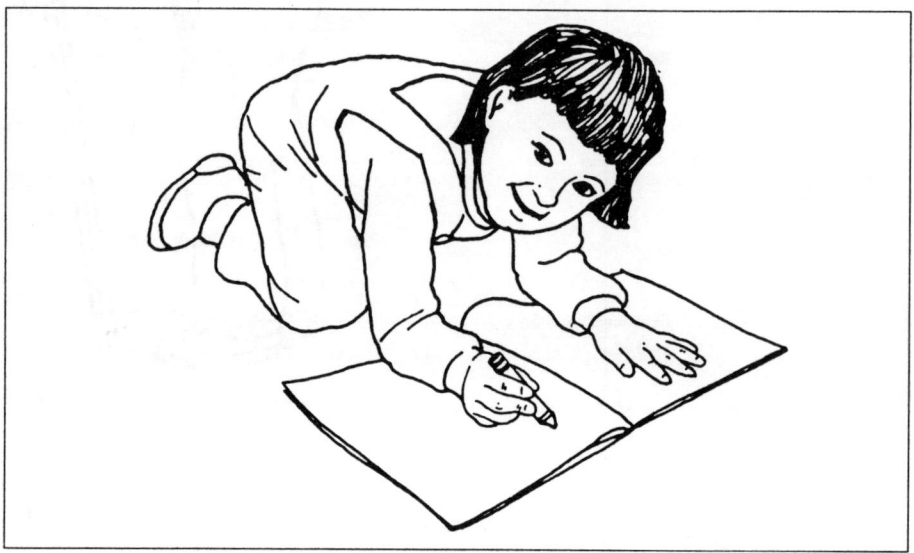

Side-Leaning

Side-leaning is another posture that puts the child on the floor and low to the ground. The child can lean on the assist-hand side and leave the lead-hand free to draw.

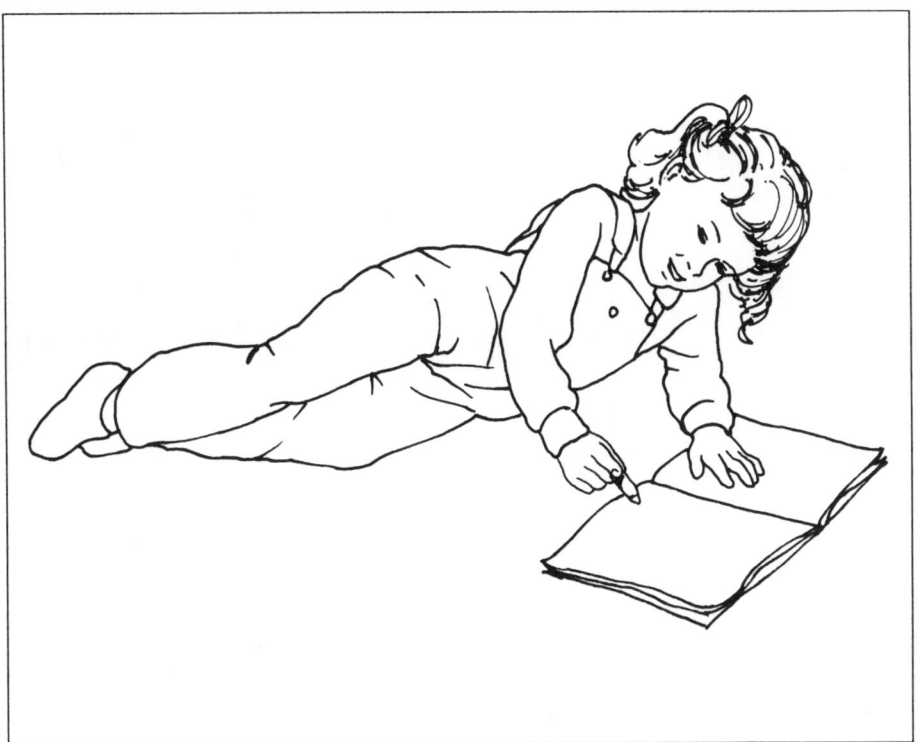

Half-Kneeling

This is one of the most challenging positions. Half-kneeling at a table is easier than without support.

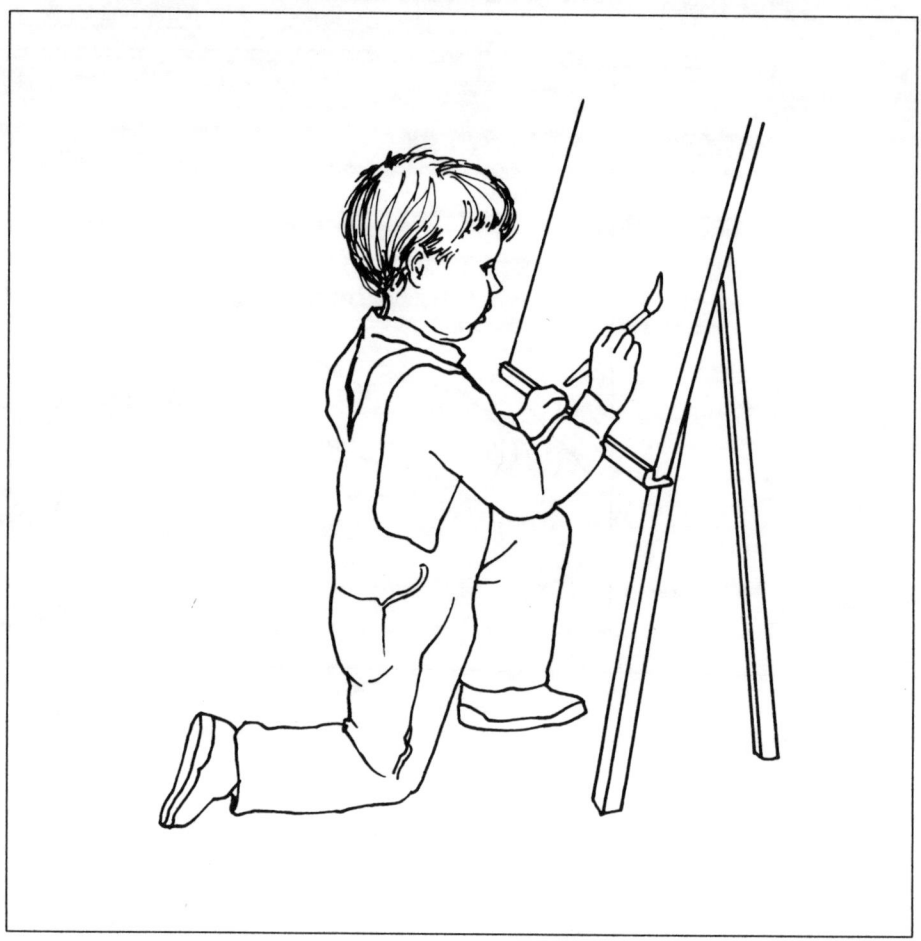

All of these practice positions can be used while the child is playing with drawing (that is, creating in a situation where anything drawn is fine). When the task has specific requirements, such as copying particular shapes, the more stable options should be chosen.

**What is a stable seating option?
When is it used?
Name two stable seating options.**

**What is a practice seating option?
When is it used?
Name five practice seating options.**

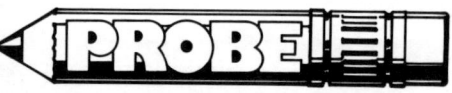

Problem Area: Poor Stability

Some children lack the shoulder, elbow, forearm, or wrist control necessary for drawing smooth, controlled lines. Their poor stability may be due to poor postural control. With better seating techniques, this problem may be eliminated or improved. The problem also may originate at the shoulder, from the child's point of proximal control, the elbow, or the wrist or hands.

■ Specific Areas of Difficulty

Shoulder Stability

Encourage the child to lean forward and rest elbows on the table or wheelchair tray. This position allows the child to use forearms, wrists, and hands from a controlled point of support at the elbows.

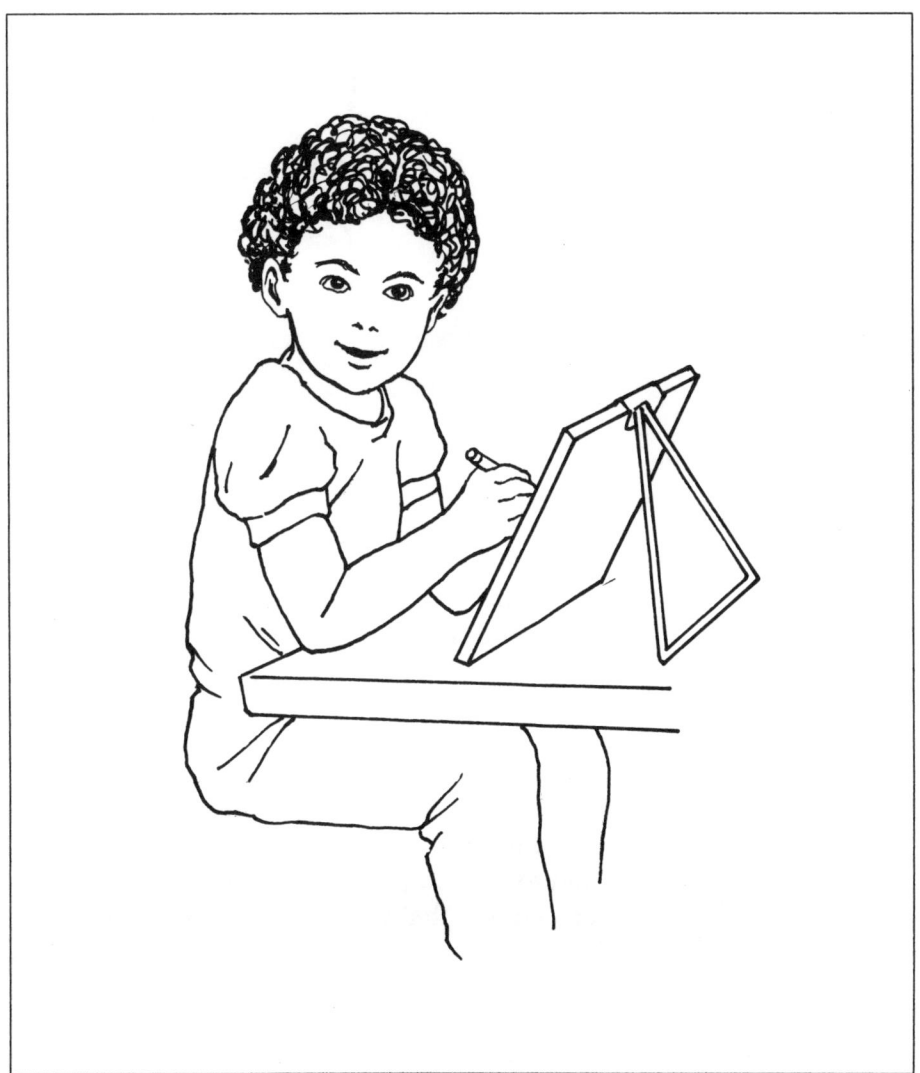

Have the child hold the upper arms at the sides of the trunk. In this position the trunk offers support, so the child does not need to control the arms away from the body at the shoulder.

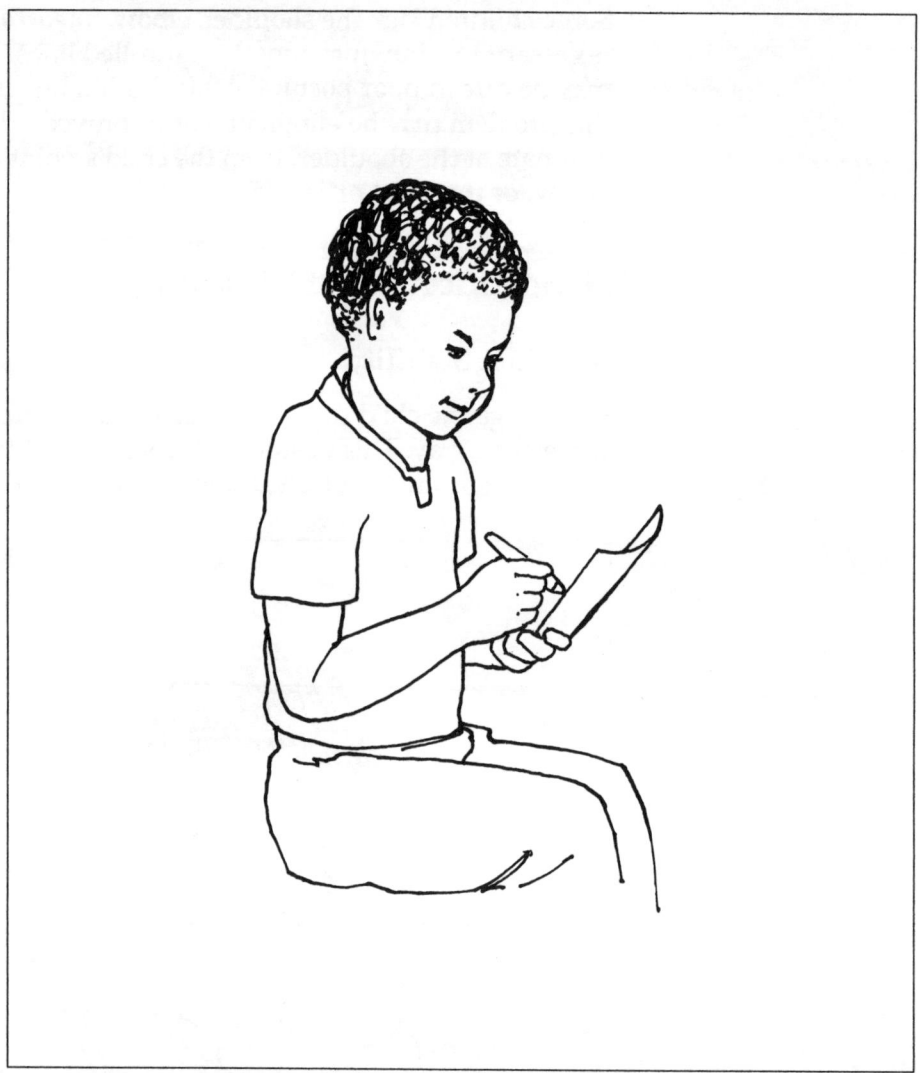

The prone or tummy-lying position (see page 46) is appropriate for improving shoulder stability. By leaning on the elbows, the child does not need to control the upper arms from the shoulder.

Elbow Stability

All of the methods used to improve shoulder stability also are appropriate for improving elbow stability. Each of those suggestions requires the child to lean on the elbows. Leaning into the joint can give it the control and stability that the child may be unable to attain independently.

Forearm Stability

Have the child lean on the desk, table, or wheelchair tray. Instead of leaning on only the elbows, the child can lean on the forearms with weight forward in the wrists.

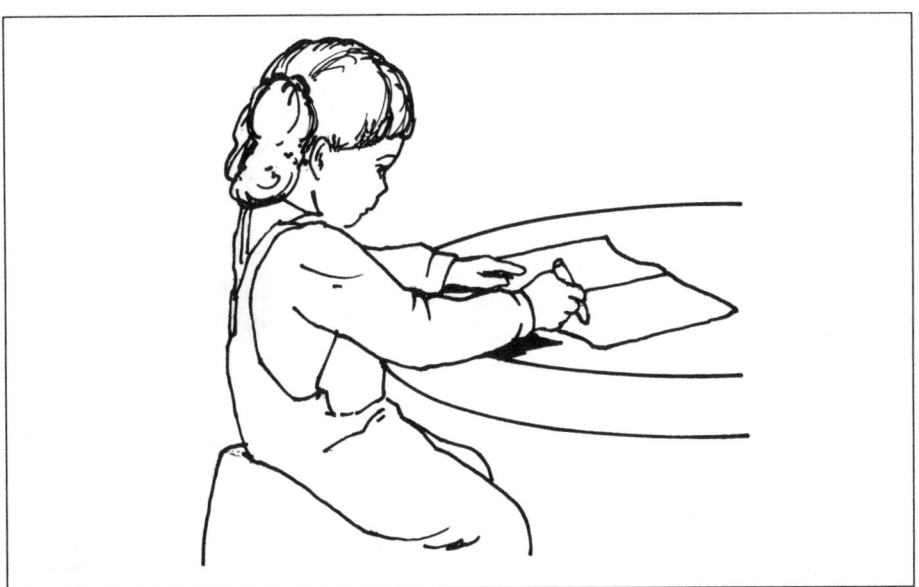

Some therapists find that having children wear 8-ounce to one-pound weights on their wrists can provide the extra proprioception or awareness of their joints to improve control.

It is important when using weights to monitor the child's progress to be sure not too much weight is used and that the weights are gradually decreased as the child gains control.

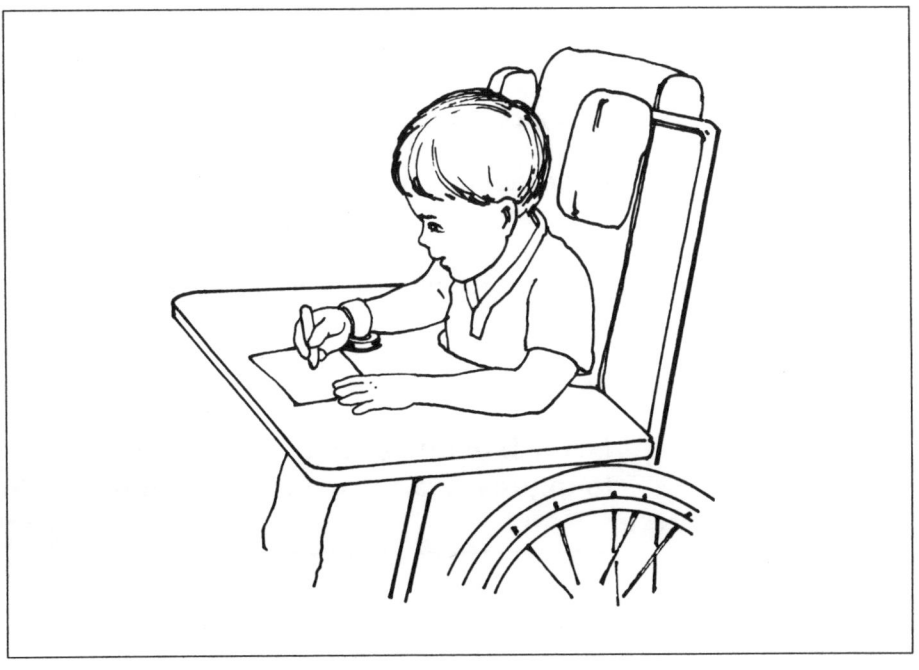

Wrist Stability

Putting weight into the wrists will help the child to gain more control at that joint. Often it is difficult to put weight into the forearm without also resting the wrist on the table. Another way to promote wrist stability is to have the child draw on a tilted board surface so that both the wrists and the forearms are resting on the surface.

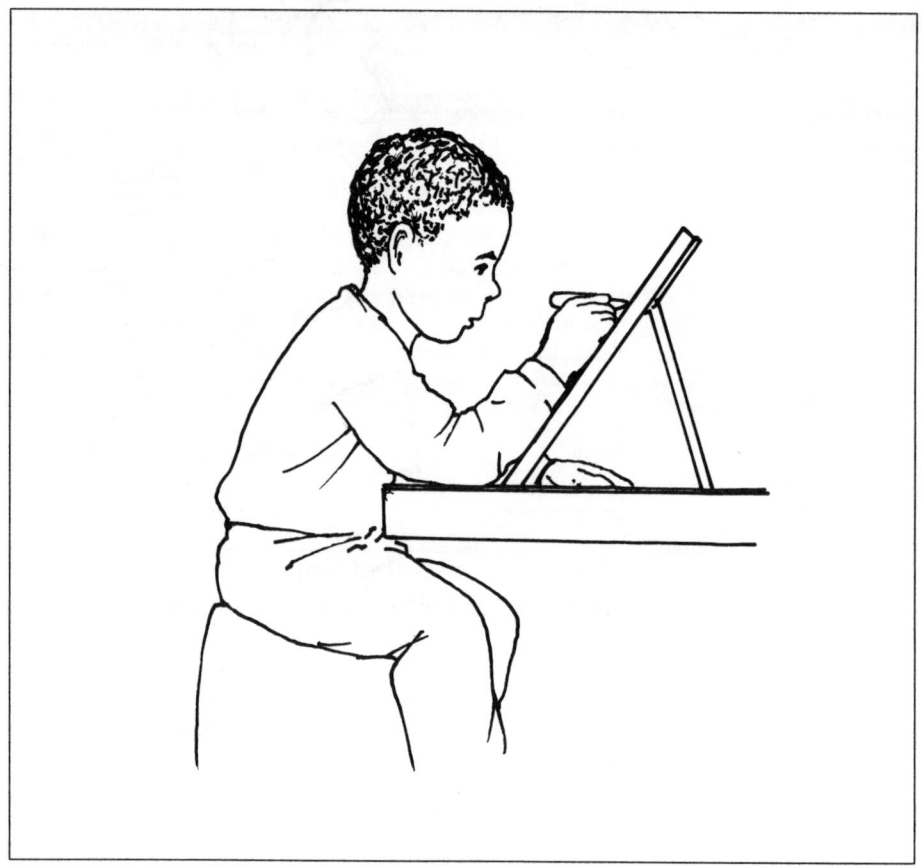

Hand Stability

Have the child rest the little-finger side of the hand on the table while using the other side of the hand to hold the writing utensil. In Chapter 6, a variety of different-shaped writing tools are described that encourage this type of hand placement.

Name five things that can be done to improve stability for pre-writing functions.

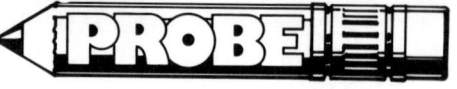

Problem Area:
Confusion about Dominance

When children begin pre-writing activities, often they are just beginning to develop a preference for leading with a particular hand. Normally it takes a child from about eighteen months to six years of age to refine the pre-writing skills necessary for writing letters with recognizable control. During that time, the child usually moves from random hand usage toward two-hand activity that requires lead and assistor patterns of movement. They have more and more experiences with fine motor activities that help them determine their hand dominance.

The use of tools in a child's play provides the opportunity to continually make choices for lead hands. Children begin to discover which hand has better control for certain activities. Spoons, forks, toothbrushes, combs, hammers, and crayons are tools that allow practice. By the time the child is five, a dominance is usually well established. A preference may appear earlier.

But some children need more time. They seem to be confused as to which hand to choose for different tool activities. One day they prefer one hand and the next day they prefer the other. They don't seem to be learning which hand has more control, and so they don't receive the experience of practice with one hand.

Initially, hand switching is acceptable and quite normal. Present the writing tool at the midline and let the child choose the hand in which to hold it. If the child's pre-writing control does not improve and switching is still prevalent as writing activities turn to diagonal lines and square, triangular, and diamond shapes, a referral to an occupational therapist may be necessary.

Describe how the use of tools influences development of hand dominance.

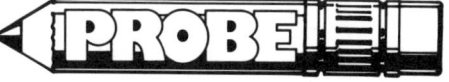

Problem Area:
Poor Lead-Assist Hand Activity

Using two hands together can be difficult for many people. This may be due to the inability to use one side of the body, as with hemiplegia or amputation, or it can be due to neurological problems, such as cerebral palsy or ataxia. The writer can stabilize the paper by taping it or by using a clipboard or notebook. Remember to place the paper at the angle necessary for a right- or left-handed person.

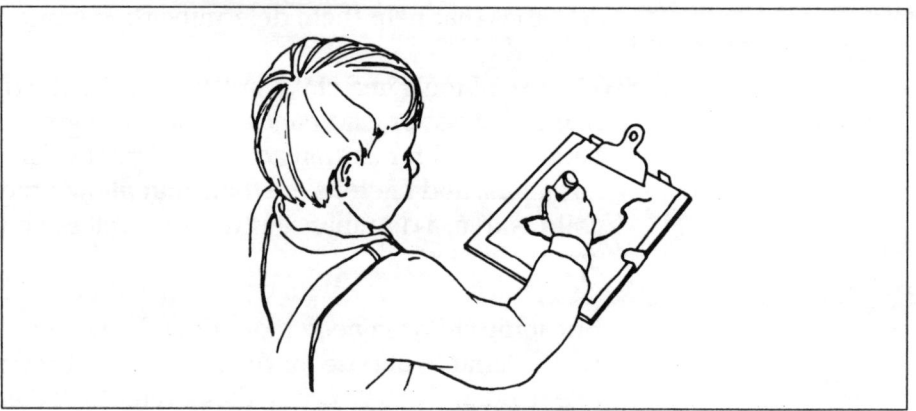

Sometimes the person has difficulty controlling the excessive movement or overflow of the nonlead hand. It may be necessary for the writer to stabilize the assist hand on a suction dowel, wheelchair arm, or drawer handle in order to keep the hand calm and reduce its interference. The writer then will need to have the paper stabilized with a clipboard or tape.

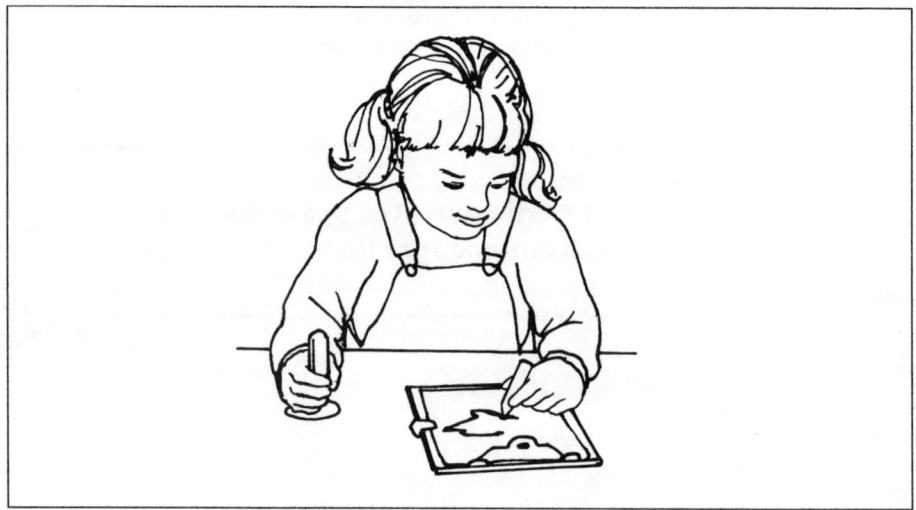

Name an activity that can assist the writer who has poor two-hand usage.

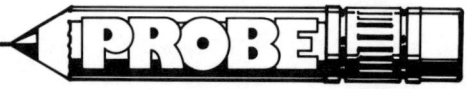

Problem Area:
Poor Grasp and Control of the Writing Tool

Many children have the cognitive abilities and the desire to learn the pre-writing sequences, but do not have the ability to grasp and control the writing tool.

If your goal is to teach the concepts of pre-writing—imitation, copying, or line direction—use a variety of activities that do not require the fine motor control of grasping a writing tool.

If your goal is to teach control of the writing tool, allow the child to practice with spontaneous drawing or with imitations of simple lines that already are known.

Do not require both pencil control and line direction imitation at first. They can be combined later as the child gains control and confidence.

■ Activities that Do Not Require Writing Tools

The concepts of imitation and copying straight, curved, intersecting, and complex lines can be taught without holding a pen or pencil. Utilize gross motor, fine motor, touch, and daily living experiences to teach pre-writing concepts. Move away from tables and chairs and leave the pens and pencils in the drawers.

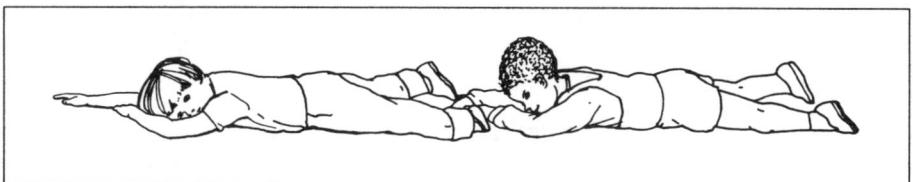

Gross Motor Activities

Have the children in your classroom be the line you are having them learn. They can lie next to each other on the floor and be vertical lines, or they can stretch out their feet to the next child's hands and be horizontal lines. They can curl up in a ball and be circles, or partially curl up and be curved lines. This activity can be done with one student or several.

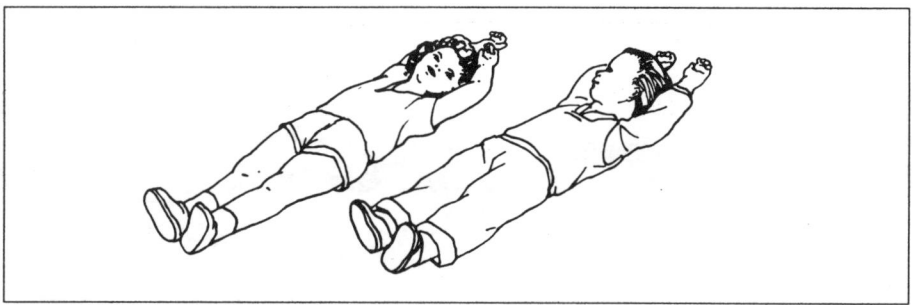

Place lines of masking tape on the floor. Children can walk, crawl, creep, hop, jump, sidestep, or skip to the table along the lines. They can wait their turn in a group activity on lines of different shapes (for example, "Wait on the curved line to go outside on the playground").

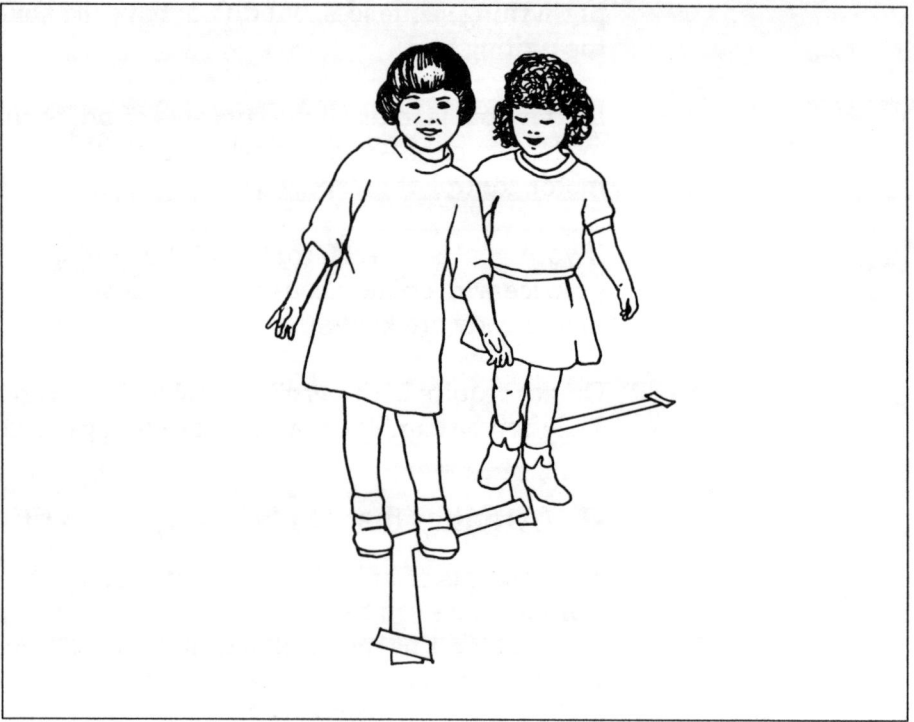

Have the children erase the chalkboard, following designated line directions. Have them clean windows or wipe tables in pre-writing directions.

The children can play with trucks and cars on sand-pile runways made in vertical, horizontal, curved, diagonal, or circular directions. Sticks can be used to make the runways.

Other gross motor activities are described in Chapters 7 and 8.

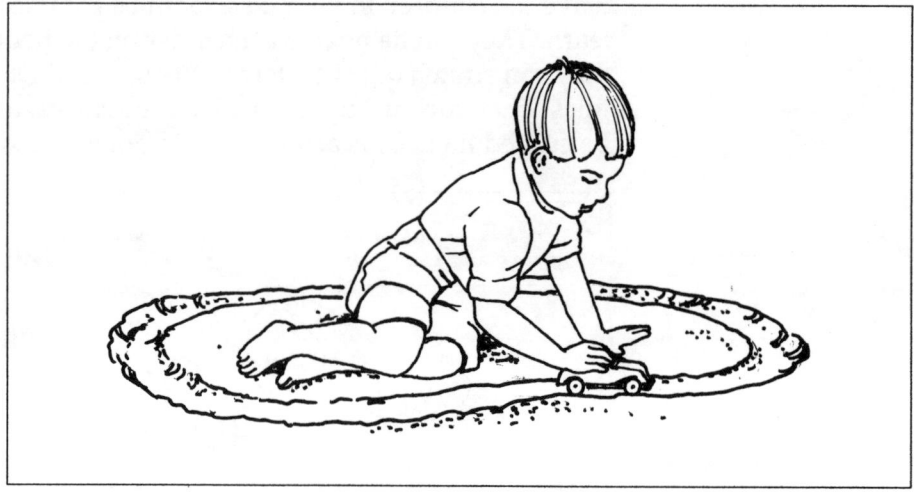

Fine Motor Activities

Many classroom activities reinforce the concepts taught in pre-writing activities. Teach those concepts throughout the day.

Blocks, sponges, paperback books, or little boxes can be stacked and knocked over. While children are learning the control and visual motor skills necessary to balance one object on top of another, they also are beginning to understand the concept of vertical direction. Blocks placed next to one another can form a train that can be pushed around the table. This activity teaches the horizontal concept.

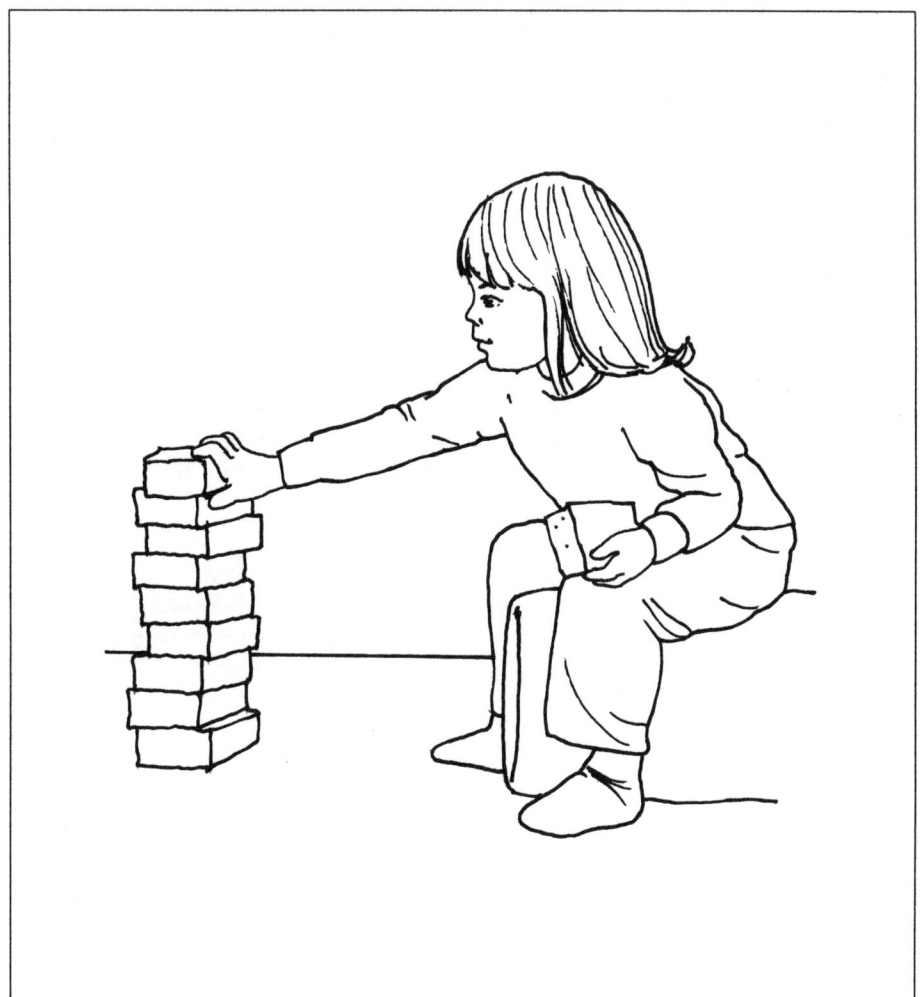

Beads can be strung to practice vertical, horizontal, and circular concepts. At the same time, the child is practicing two-handed control and lead-assist activities.

Use your imagination! By looking around the classroom and *thinking pre-writing*, you will come up with more activities!

Sensory Activities

Sometimes we can get stuck in using the same activities over and over. There are so many ways to practice the pre-writing concepts without pens and pencils. Many of those ways provide the opportunity for the children to feel different textures and sensations. Finger painting can be done with paints, powders, and lotions. Drawing can be done in sand or mud or on cakes with frosting or confectioner's sugar.

Tracing can be done with hands or fingertips on yarn, sandpaper, or holes punched in paper.

Chapter 4 contains other suggestions to promote sensory experiences for vision, touch, hearing, smell, taste, and proprioceptive movement.

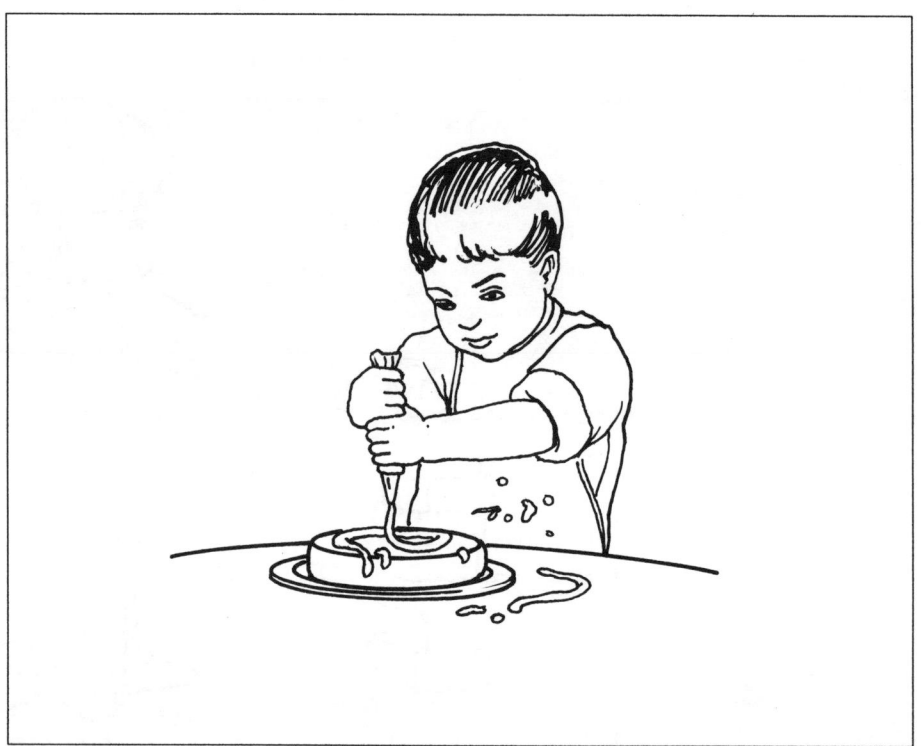

Daily Living Activities

Use lines during dressing and mealtime activities. Snaps, buttons, and zippers can help the child practice the up-and-down motions necessary for making vertical lines in pre-writing activities. Point out that clothing is put away horizontally in piles in drawers or in vertical lines next to each other in closets.

Cookies and cakes can be decorated with vertical, horizontal, diagonal, or circular designs. They can be made in circles, squares, rectangles, and other shapes. A "line" of liquid is created in pouring. A sandwich can be cut with straight or diagonal lines.

Look around, and you will find lines and shapes everywhere!

■ Using Writing Tools

What do you do when you have been practicing the pre-writing concepts without pens and pencils for a while and you cannot avoid the writing utensils any longer? Children may need to use different types of pens and pencils. The writing tools may have to be bigger than usual. They may need to be specially shaped. Some children may need help in keeping the pencil in their hands. See Chapter 6 for discussion of various types of writing tools and the situations for which they can be used.

**For each of the following categories,
list a pre-writing activity that does not require usual writing tools:**

**Gross motor activities
Fine motor activities
Sensory activities
Daily living activities**

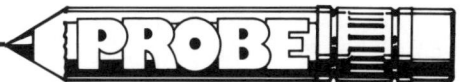

Problem Area:
Difficulty in Moving from an Immature to a Mature Grasp

Some people persist in holding the pencil as one would hold a bicycle handle. All fingers are doing the same thing at the same time with the thumb held on the opposite side on the pencil. The drawing is done with the hand held in a palm-down position or in a thumb-down position. Both positions are inefficient for precise writing control.

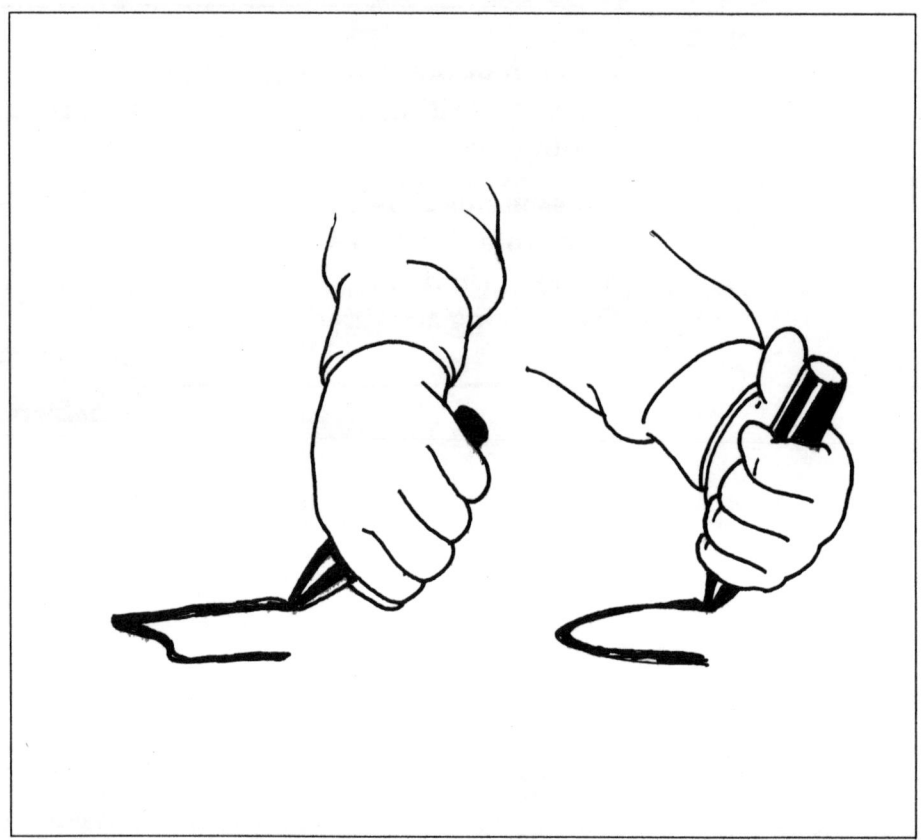

Triangular-shaped pens, pencils, and crayons can be used to facilitate a more mature grasp. The sides provide three separate surfaces to hold. This provides the cues and feedback necessary for more successful pencil holding.

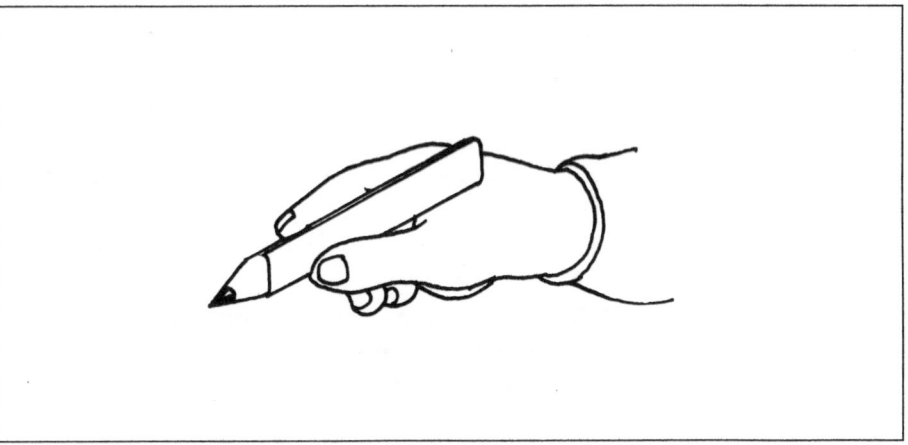

Triangular-shaped pencil grips also encourage a mature grasp.

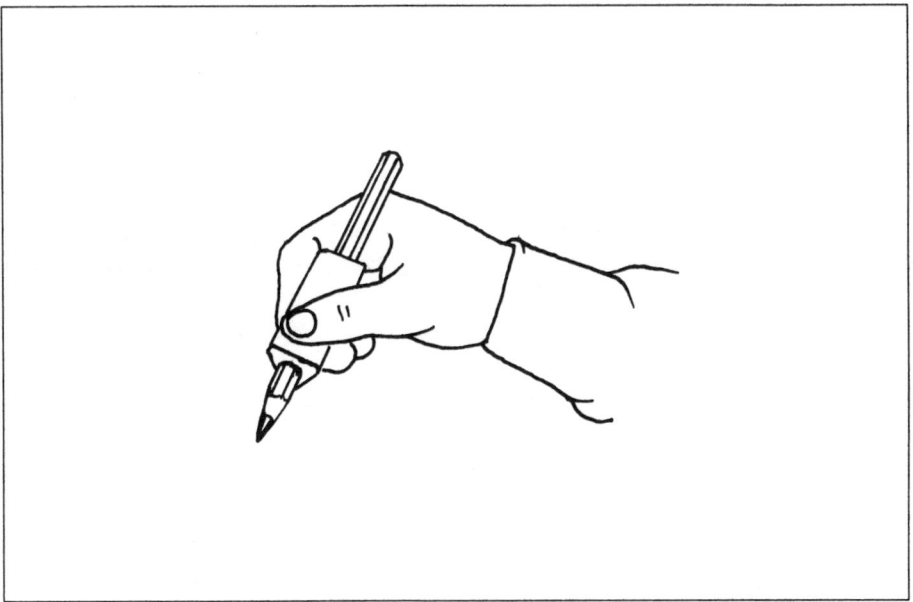

Name two options that may assist in moving from an immature to a mature grasp.

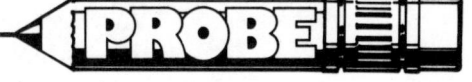

Problem Area: Poor Attention Span

Students demonstrate poor attention span for a number of reasons. Perhaps they are bored or hungry. The task may be too difficult. Or the problem may be caused by distractibility or hyperactivity.

If the student is bored, the activity can be changed and made more fun. If the student is hungry, a snack can be given, or the pre-writing tasks can be presented after lunch rather than before. If the presentation is too difficult, the teacher needs to review the student's skills to be sure the lesson is appropriate to the student's developmental level.

Distractibility and hyperactivity are more complicated to understand. It is important to create the lesson plan so the student's attention is focused on the pre-writing task rather than on the environment. Sometimes distractibility can be eliminated just by having the task be so exciting that the student's attention is drawn to the task.

■ Involving the Senses

Consider all the sensory variables.

Vision

Use vision to draw the student's attention to the task, not away from it. Use brightly colored markers, finger paints, and papers. Try to eliminate distracting peripheral visual movements, such as other students walking by. Some children may need to learn the new parts of the pre-writing sequence in a cubbie corner away from classroom visual distractions.

Hearing

The sounds the children hear may take away their attention. Music in the room or the clanking of lunch preparation in a nearby kitchen may be too much distraction for some children. Sound can be added to the task in front of the child. Bells can be put on pens. Paper placed on sandpaper creates a different noise when the student is drawing. A Talking Pen is described on page 74. This electronic pen-and-paper system uses a fiber-optic sensor to pick up reflected light. It buzzes as the writer traces lines appropriately.

Touch

Varying the touch or tactile aspects of the pre-writing activity can draw the student's attention to the task. Finger paints, powders, and soap lather can be great fun for pre-writing tasks. Change the place mat on which the student draws. By placing the paper on textured fabric or paper, the student will experience different sensations while drawing. Corduroy or nubby fabric will be much different from sandpaper when marking lines or circles.

Taste

It certainly will bring a student's attention to the task if finger painting is done with whipped cream or chocolate pudding or yogurt that can be tasted!

Smell

Markers now come in many fragrances that are wonderful attention getters.

■ Posture and Movement

Remember that the student's attention should not focus on an uncomfortable position. This is why it is so important to think about positioning and seating before presenting a pre-writing task.

How can you help students who have a very difficult time sitting still—those students who fidget and wiggle and always have to move? Can you incorporate movement into the activity rather than creating a stationary task? Have the students roll to the pencil box and then crawl to the paper. Or have them stand around a table and make a group picture on a table covered with butcher paper. Or have them take giant steps to the easel, draw, and then walk sideways to their seats.

■ Referral

Even with creative lesson planning and individualized assistance, some students still will have difficulty in attending to the tasks presented. If the problem persists, a referral to a perceptual-motor specialist (such as an occupational or physical therapist) or a developmental psychologist may be necessary.

List six ways to vary sensory aspects of the pre-writing task to help students improve their attention span.

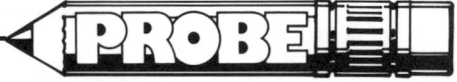

Problem Area:
Poor Imitation Skills

Some students have difficulty imitating the lines and shapes that are presented. Be sure the tasks are developmentally appropriate for that particular student. Try presenting the concept using a variety of different sensory activities. Use whole-body games and fine-motor imitations. Use templates. Students can feel the shape on the template with fingers, hands, or even elbows and feet. They can trace the lines on yarn, fabric, sandpaper, or in dirt. They can do it with their eyes open and closed.

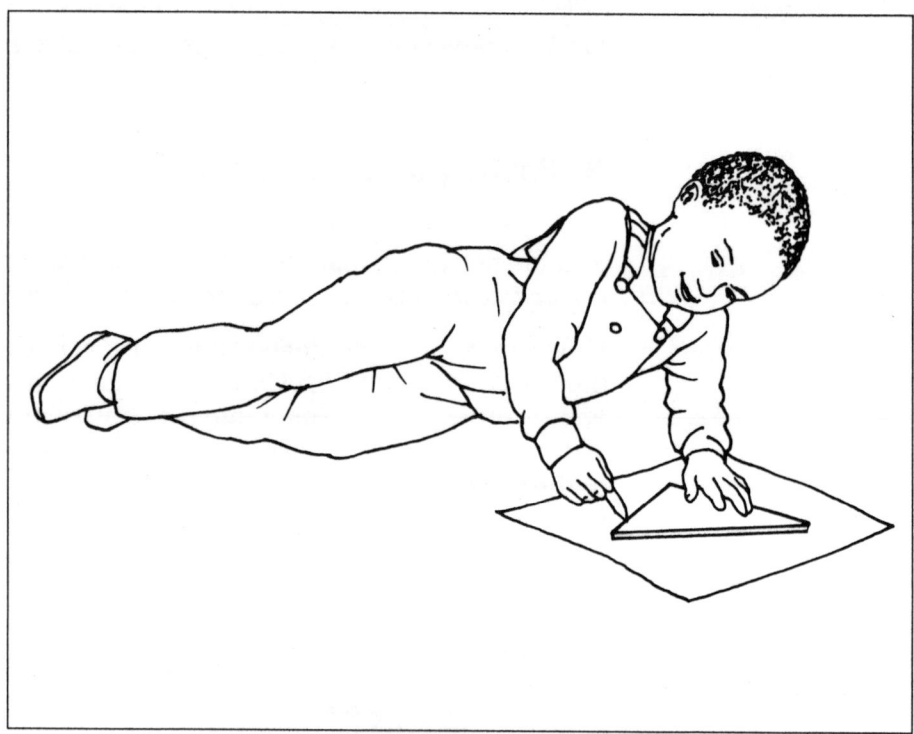

Some students may be able to imitate horizontal, vertical, and even circular lines quite well; and problems may not arise until the task requires diagonals, intersecting lines, and production of recognizable shapes. It is quite common for students with some difficulties in the more refined aspects of motor planning not to demonstrate their problems until more complex demands are placed on them. A referral to a specialist may be necessary for children who have persistent problems in this area.

Describe two ways to increase sensory information in an imitation activity.

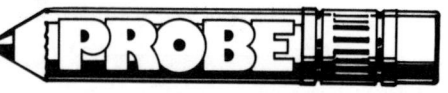

Problem Area: Limited Vision

People who have visual limitations may need extra assistance to succeed at pre-writing activities. Individuals with some vision may need to use pens that are highly contrasting to the paper color. The paper also may need to contrast sharply with the table color. Extra tactile cues may be important for providing the feedback normally received through vision. Templates help provide information on where to draw.

Tracing also can help those with limited vision to feel the direction and shapes. Use yarn, sandpaper, hole-punched lines, or string to highlight the shape to be drawn. Help the person to feel the shape with hands or, preferably, fingertips before attempting to draw the shape itself.

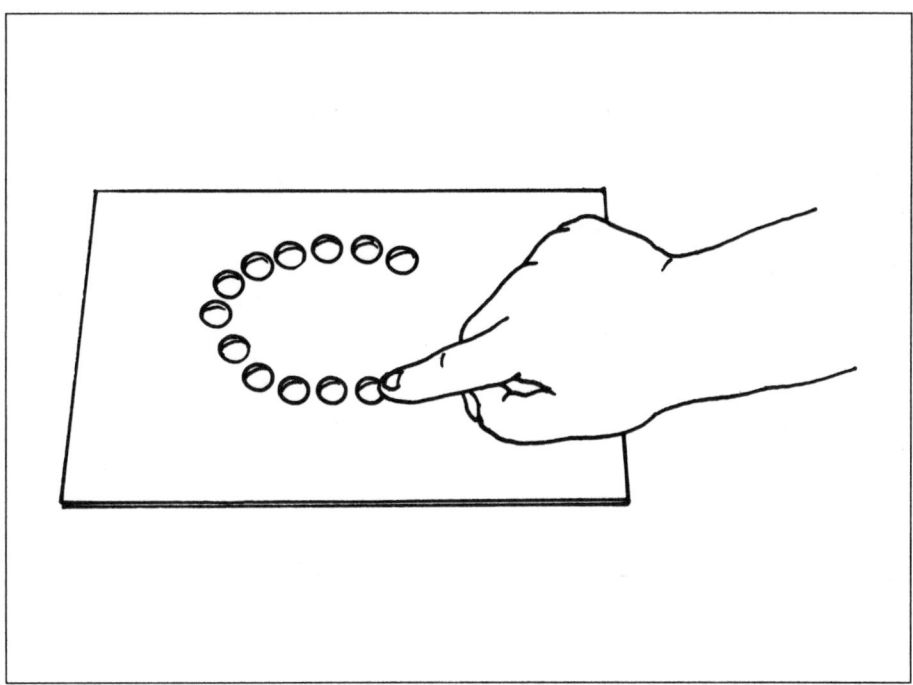

Sighted people's vision provides feedback about what was just drawn. We need to think of creative ways for those with limited vision to receive this feedback. For example, drawing in clay, sand, or cookie dough can provide a groove that provides that kind of information.

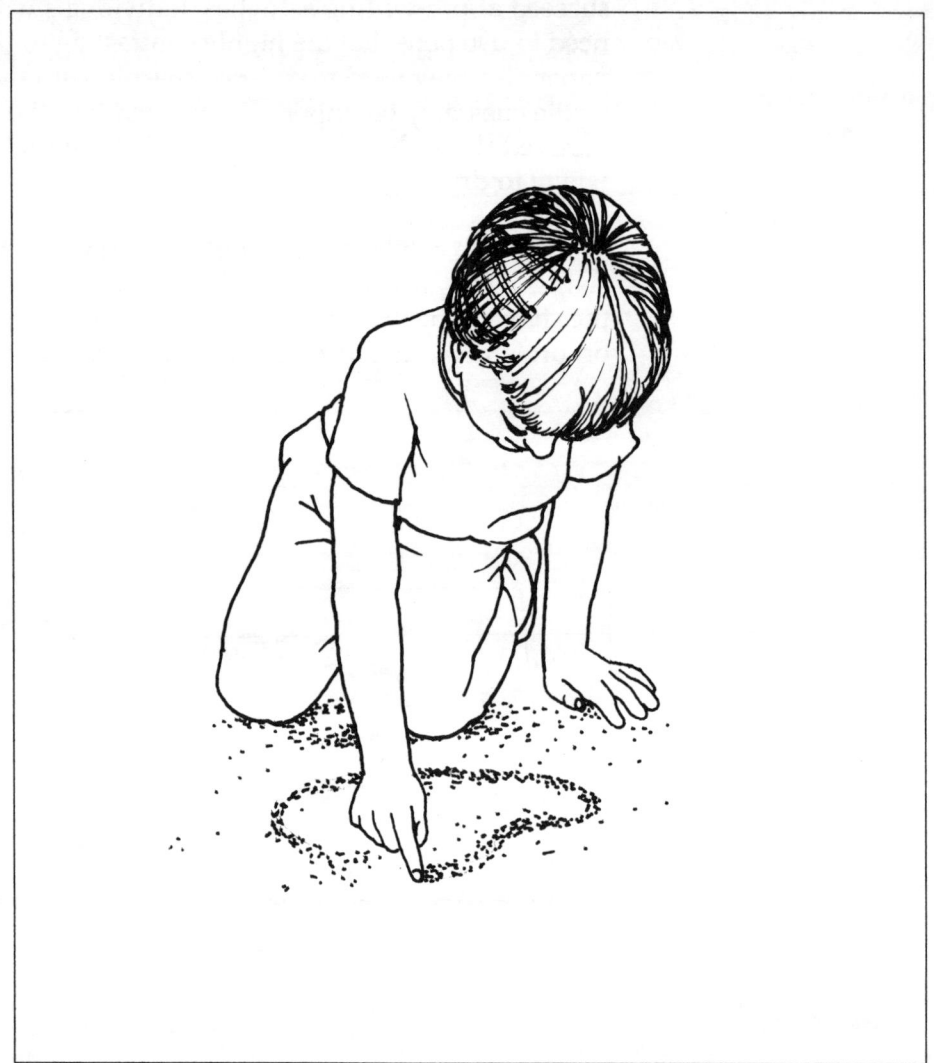

Describe two ways to provide sensory information for children with limited vision.

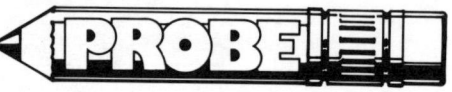

Problem Area: Inability to Use Hands

Those who have extremely poor ability to control the muscles of the upper extremities and people with congenital or traumatic amputation of both arms will need to find another way to perform fine motor tasks. Head pointers or mouth sticks can be used as the extra limb for this type of function. A marking pen can be attached to the pointer so the person can make the marks by moving the head.

When first providing the opportunity for drawing with a head pointer, allow plenty of time for practice with random marks. Do not start by having the person imitate or copy your marks. As with any instruction on writing, the student needs time just to become familiar with the task and learn how to make the pointer or marker work.

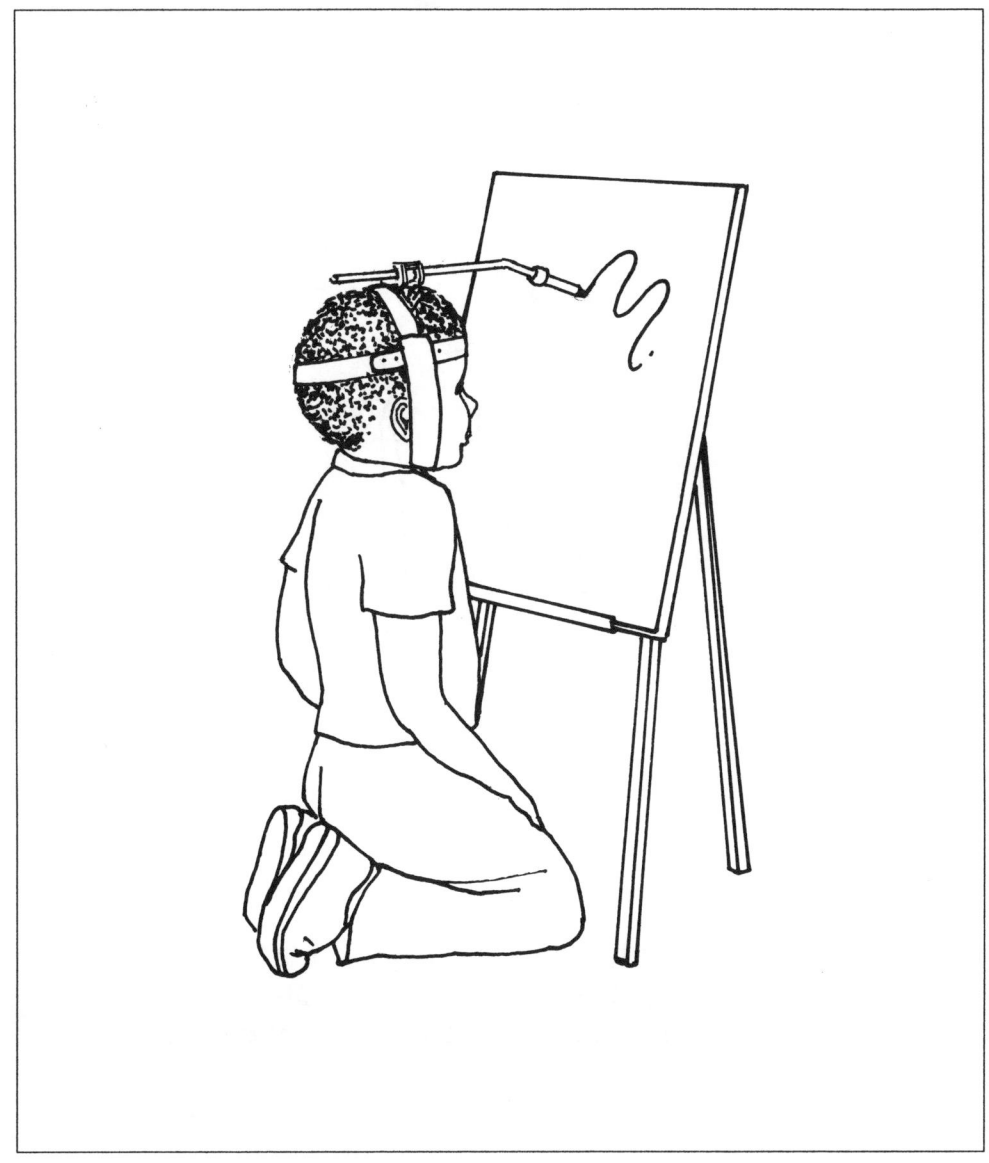

A different way to help the student practice is to darken the room and attach a penlight flashlight to the pointer. Let the student "draw" with the light. The student can draw all over the room, find certain objects with the light, or make "spaceships" on the walls. Tape a large sheet of butcher paper to the wall and take a marking pen in your hand. As the student "draws" with the light, trace the pattern on the paper.

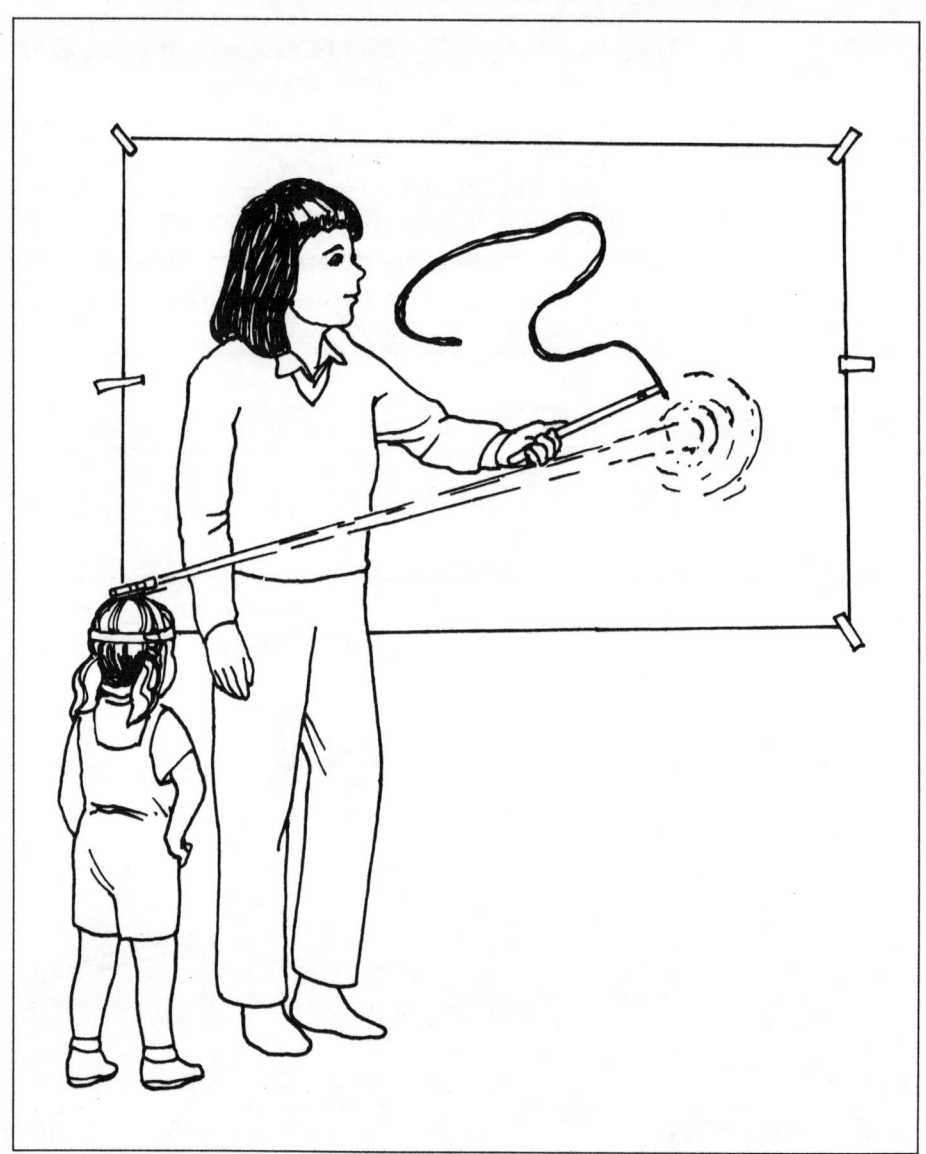

Name two ways for students to practice pre-writing concepts when they do not have functional use of their hands.

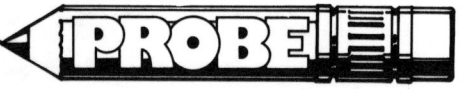

6 Adaptive Pre-Writing Equipment

Many different commercially manufactured or homemade pieces of adaptive pre-writing equipment are described in this chapter. This area of expertise is constantly changing, and this list may not include all equipment currently available. Please note that no one distributor is recommended over another and that the list may not include all distributors of each piece of equipment. Distributors' addresses are listed on page 82.

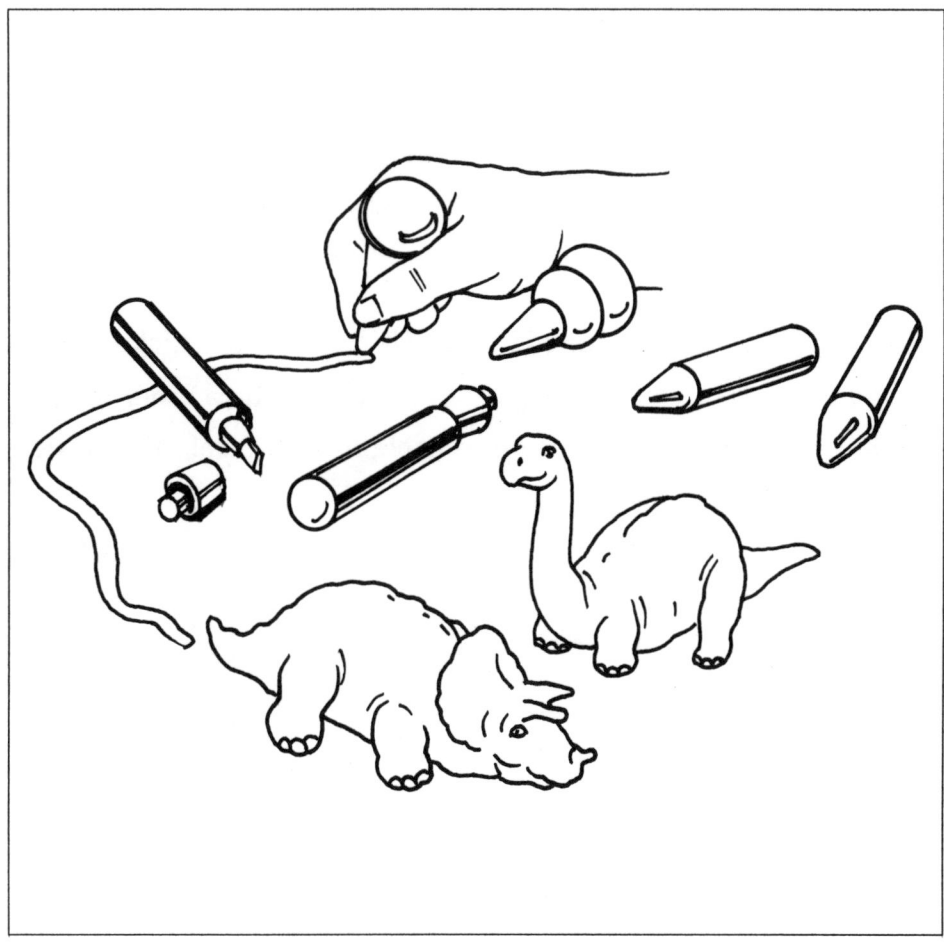

■ Thick Chalks

Short, thick chalks fit well into little fingers. A child can use a whole-hand grasp easily.

Distributors Thick chalks are manufactured by several companies. They have different names and slightly different shapes or packaging but are all similar. They are available in most teaching supply stores and children's and toy shops, or they can be ordered from:

Teaching Resources

Childcraft Education Corporation

Lakeshore Curriculum Materials

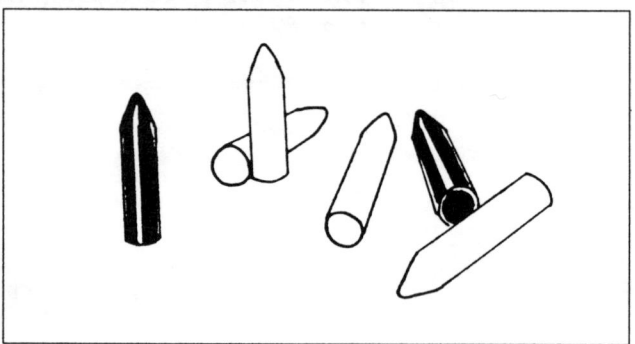

■ Large Markers, Thick Pencils, Thick Crayons

Large writing tools are easier for little hands to hold.

Distributors These items are available in most school, office, variety, and children's stores.

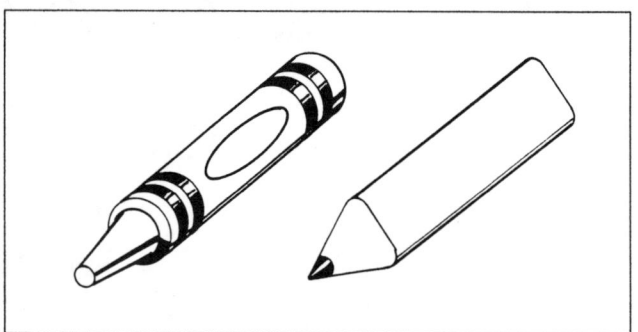

■ Square Crayons

These crayons are short and wide and fit into a little hand. A mature grasp is not required; a whole-hand grasp can be used.

Distributors These crayons are manufactured and distributed by several companies and have different names. They are available in school supply and children's stores, or they can be ordered from:

Teaching Tools

Lakeshore Curriculum Materials

Childcraft Education Corporation

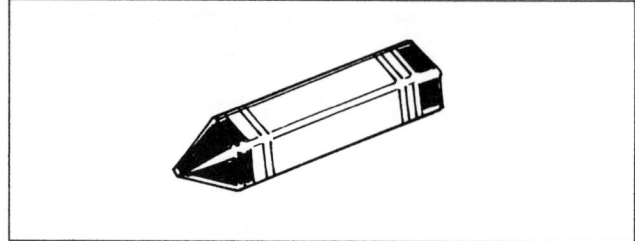

■ Easy-Grip Crayons

The unusual design of these crayons makes it easier for little hands to control them. They can be held with a whole-hand grasp with palm down, or they can be used to facilitate a beginning mature grasp because of the special index-finger indentation. These crayons have become very popular at preschools around the country.

Distributors   Easy-grip crayons can be purchased at most variety and school supply stores.

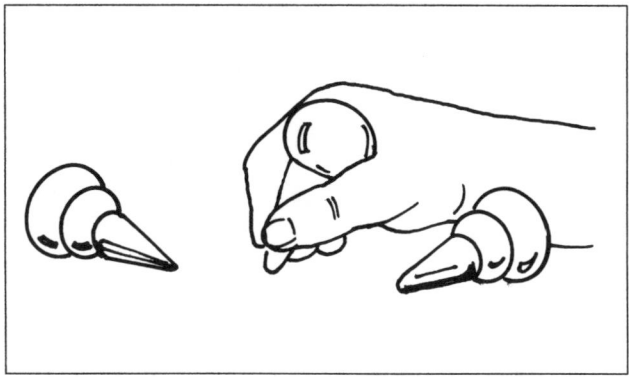

■ Scented Markers

These markers come in many scents. They are used successfully to keep a child's attention on pre-writing tasks.

Distributors   These are available in most variety stores.

■ Decorator Crayons

These crayons are designed especially for children. They come in a variety of different shapes, including dinosaurs, farm animals, fruits, or vehicles. Usually they are short and wide, a design that fits well into young hands. They are fun and are good attention getters.

Distributors   These crayons are available in toy and variety stores.

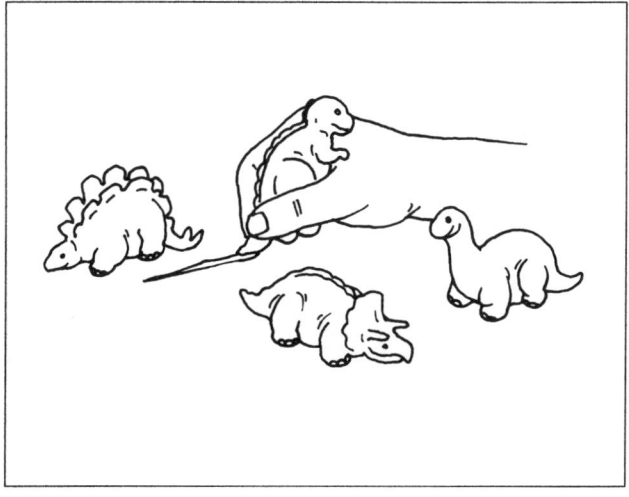

■ **Easy-Bend Pens**

These pens are designed for children. They are wider than an average pen. Children can hold the end and wrap the bendable handle around their hand. These pens can be used to facilitate a more mature grasp.

Distributors These are available in variety and toy stores.

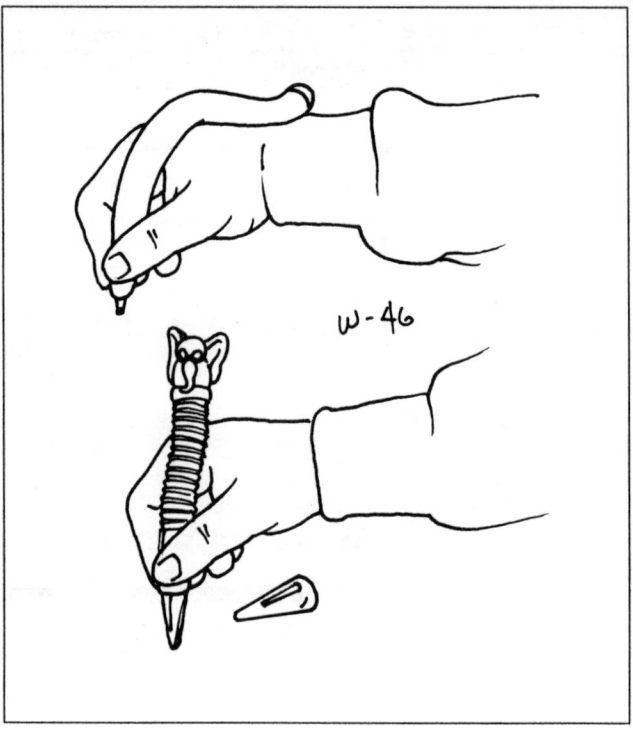

■ **Talking Pen™**

This electronic pen has a small beam of light on its infrared tip. When the tip is on a colored surface, a sensor picks up the reflected light and causes a buzzer to sound. The continuous buzz when tracing provides audibility to the writer.

Manufactured and distributed by Wayne Engineering

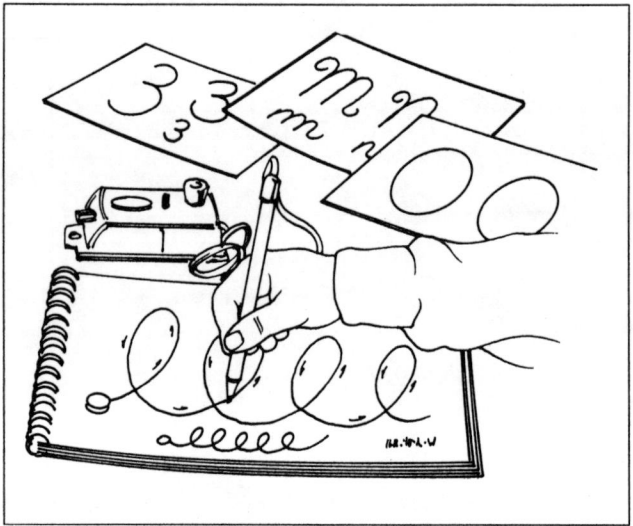

■ Pencil Grips

These pencil grips are an excellent tool to help a person redirect an immature pencil grasp to a more mature one. The three sides of the grip guide the thumb, index finger, and middle finger into the appropriate position.

Distributors These are available at most office and school supply stores.

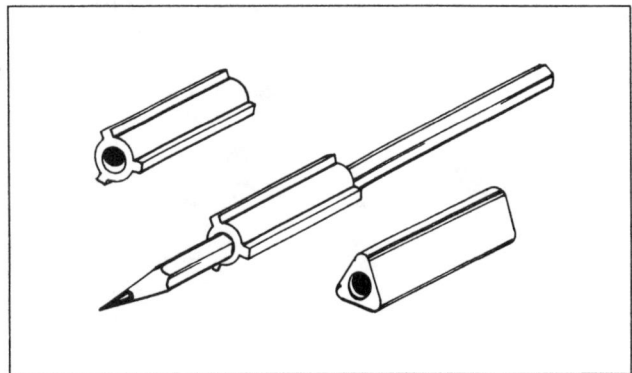

■ My-Grip™ Personal Grips

These are customized pencil grips made of cylindrical tubing that can be cut to the appropriate size. Put them in hot water, then mold them to the appropriate pincer shape.

Distributor Fred Sammons, Inc.

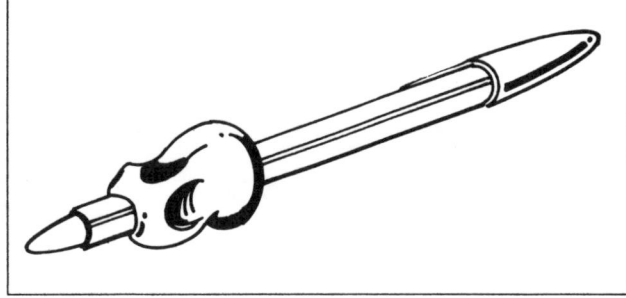

■ Stethro™ Pencil Holders

This holder fits on a pencil. Its shape is designed for placing the index and middle fingers and thumb in a comfortable, mature grasp for writing.

Distributors These pencil holders are available at most office and school supply stores.

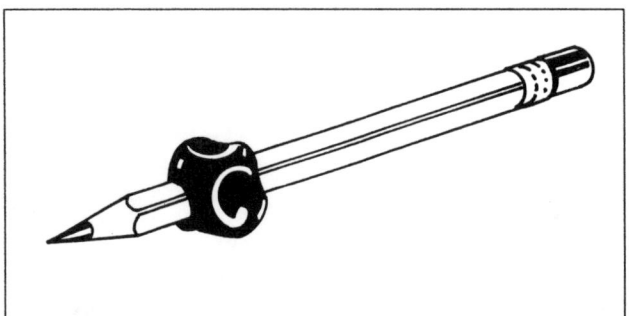

■ Triangular Pencils, Crayons

These writing tools facilitate a more mature grasp by guiding placement of the thumb and index and middle fingers. They are made wider than the average crayon or pencil to make grasping easier for young or unstable hands.

Distributors These are available in many school and office supply stores, or they can be ordered from:

Constructive Play Things

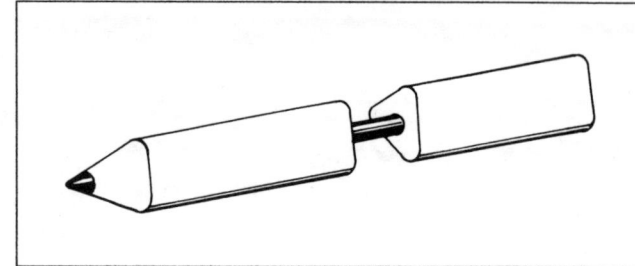

■ Weighted Pens

This pen is weighted with 8- to 10-gram weights. The extra weight can be a great assistance for hands that are slightly shaky.

Distributor Fred Sammons, Inc.

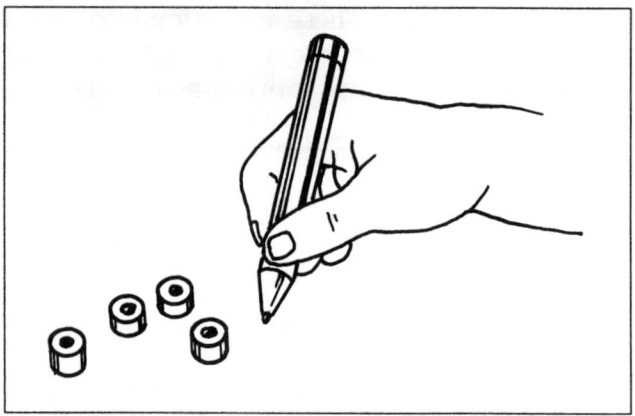

■ Cylindrical Foam Padding

This foam padding can be cut to the desired length and placed around a crayon or pen to enlarge the handle for easier handling.

Distributors Help Yourself Aids

Medical Equipment Distributors

Fred Sammons, Inc.

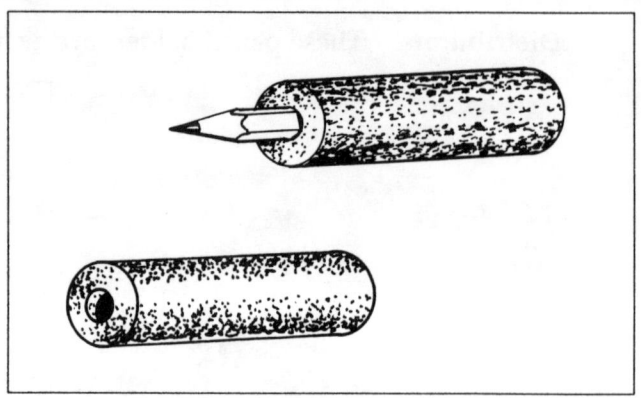

■ Built-Up Handle

This sturdy wooden handle can be used to enlarge the handle of crayons, pens, markers, paintbrushes, and pencils. It is an excellent choice for adolescents and adults who need the assistance of a larger handle.

Distributors Help Yourself Aids

Medical Equipment Distributors

Fred Sammons, Inc.

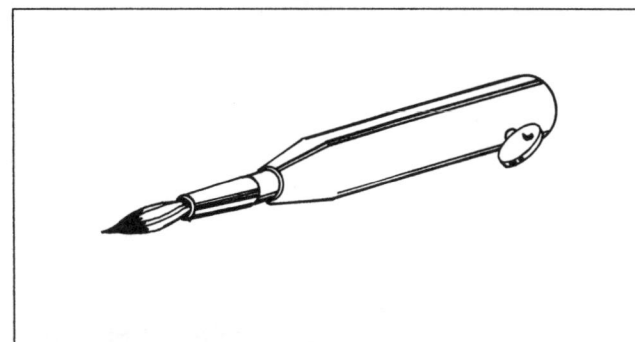

■ Universal Cuff

This hand cuff provides support for the writing tool. It is useful for those who have difficulty maintaining the necessary grasp for writing.

Distributors Help Yourself Aids

Medical Equipment Distributors

Fred Sammons, Inc.

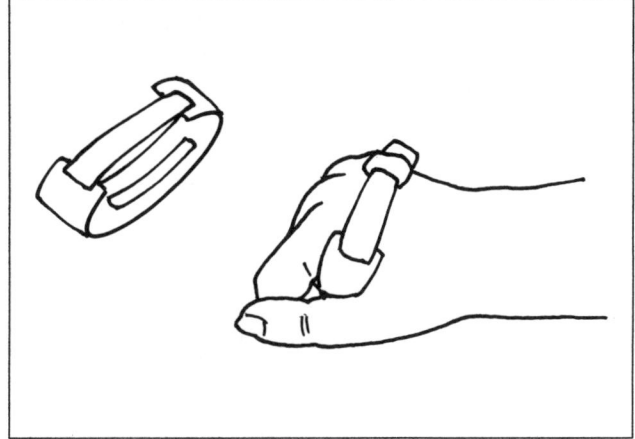

■ Extension Holder or Right-Angle Double Pocket

This device has two pockets to hold pens or pencils. The handle of the writing tool is held in the hand.

Distributors Fred Sammons, Inc.

Medical Equipment Distributors

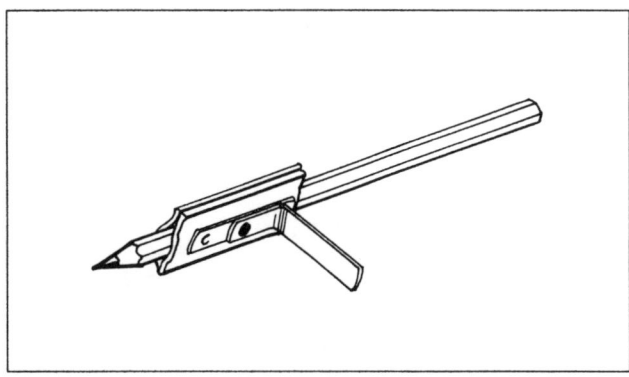

■ Klik ™ Pencil Holder

This holder circles the hand. Its side rollers hold a pen or marker in place for writing.

Distributors Fred Sammons, Inc.

Help Yourself Aids

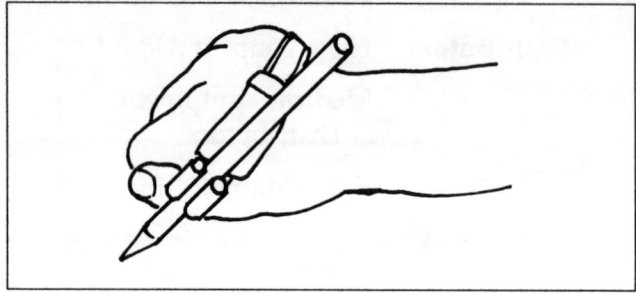

■ Sarong Pencil Holder

With this sarong, the hand is held in the appropriate position for a mature grasp. This holder is designed for adults.

Distributors Fred Sammons, Inc.

Help Yourself Aids

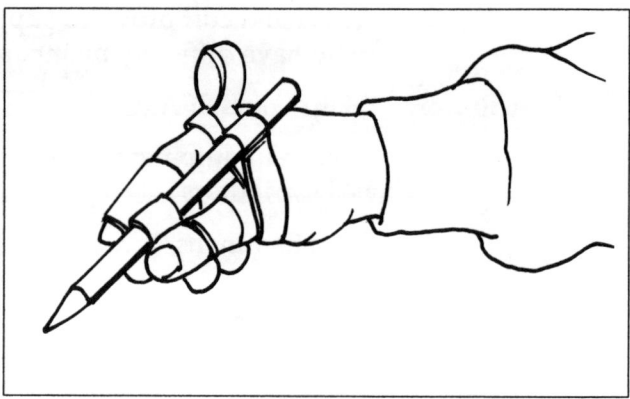

■ Writing Frame

This bow-shaped wire frame holds the pencil upright for writing. The person must have finger action to hold the pencil, but the rest of the hand is supported by the tripod. This frame is designed for adults.

Distributors Fred Sammons, Inc.

Help Yourself Aids

Medical Equipment Distributors

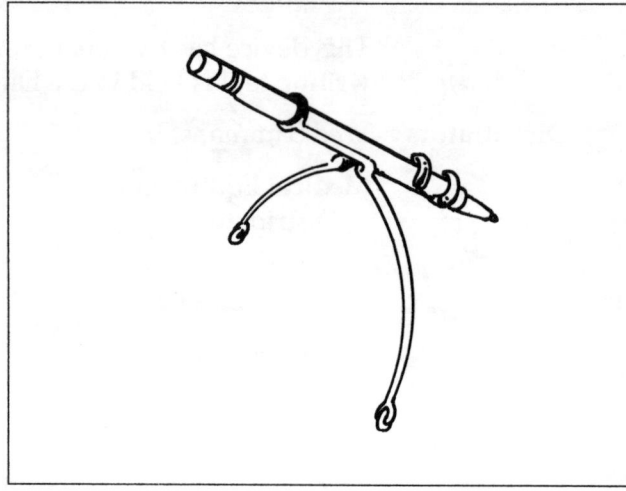

■ Slip-On Writing Aid

This holder is contoured to hold a pen securely in the hand while providing an adjustable angle for writing. Adjustments are made with a heat gun. It is designed for adults and must be purchased specifically for the left or right hand.

Distributor   Fred Sammons, Inc.

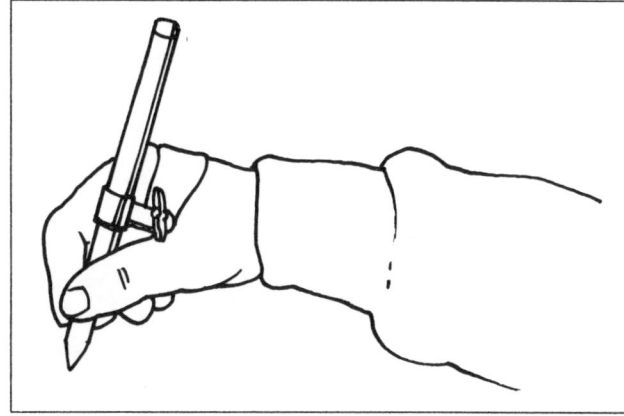

■ Wanchik Writer ™

This holder keeps the palm and fingers in the appropriate position for writing.

Distributor   Fred Sammons, Inc.

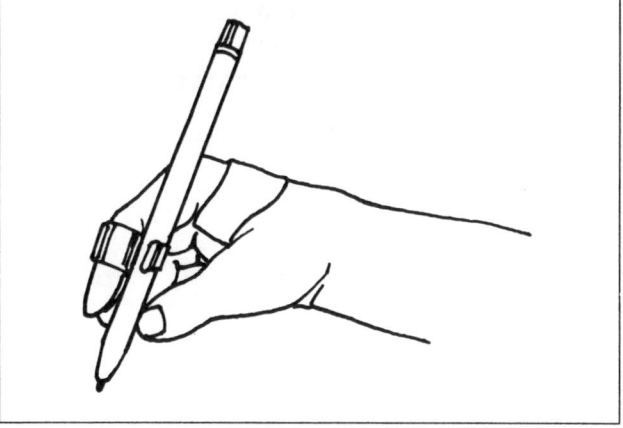

■ Wanchik Writer #2 ™

This plastic-covered metal splint or orthosis is designed to provide the wrist support necessary for writing.

Distributor   Fred Sammons, Inc.

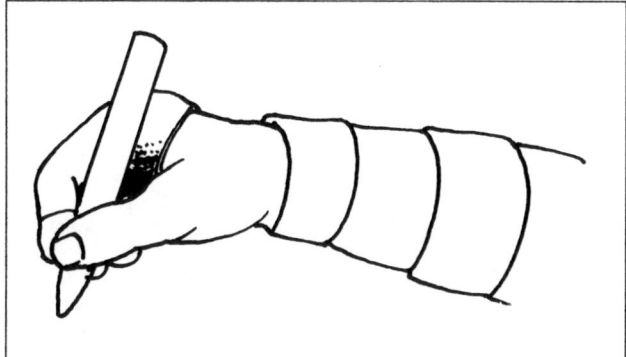

■ One-Handed Writing Board

This writing board has a lever that allows the writer to position the paper. Rubber stoppers on the bottom keep the board from moving.

Distributors Fred Sammons, Inc.

Help Yourself Aids

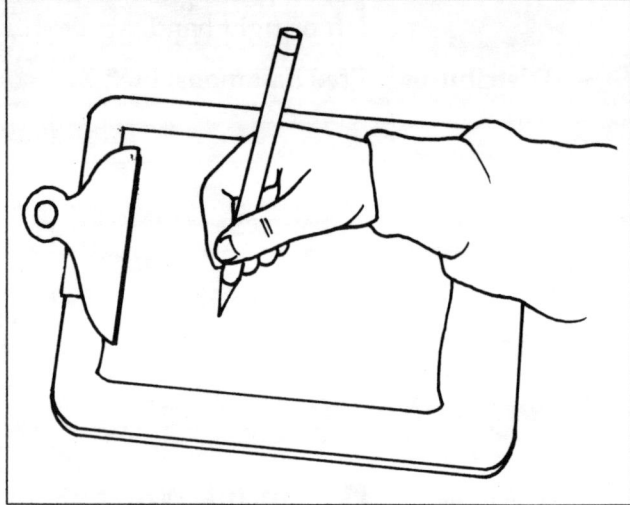

■ Wrist Hold-Down

This magnet is designed to stabilize the hand and wrist. A 12" x 18" metal plate and three magnet cuffs allow the user to vary the amount of resistance offered by the magnet.

Distributor Fred Sammons, Inc.

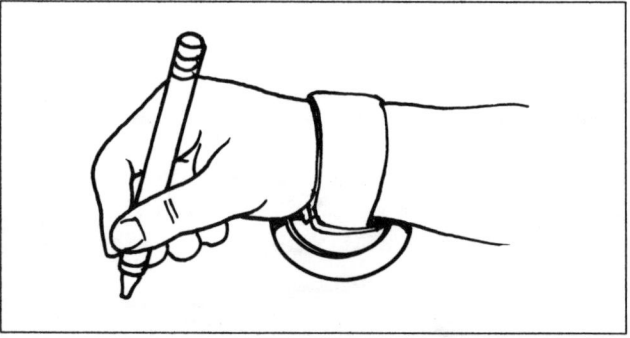

■ Suction Dowel

This dowel has a suction base that is designed to stay where placed on a table. The writer holds the dowel to stabilize that hand or side of the body.

Distributor Fred Sammons, Inc.

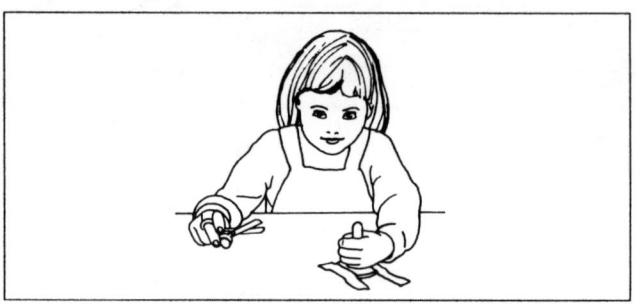

■ Head Pointer

The head pointer is used by individuals who have difficulty functioning adequately with their hands. Writing utensils are controlled by head movements instead of hands.

Distributors   Adaptive Theraputic Systems, Inc.

Medical Equipment Distributors

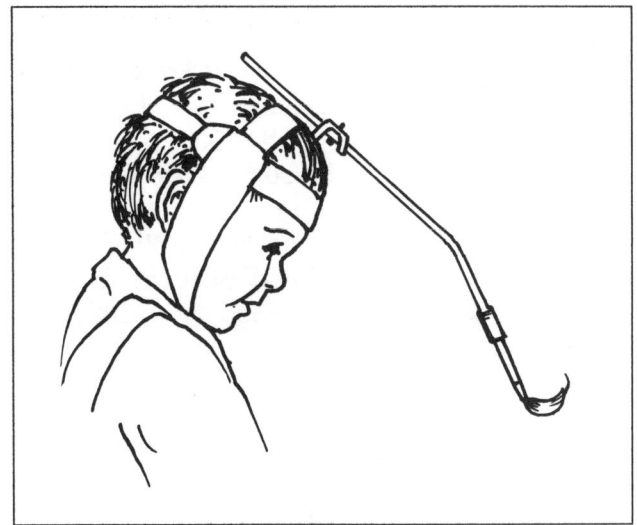

■ Mouth Stick

The mouth stick can be used to control writing implements when hands are unable to be used.

Distributor   Medical Equipment Distributors

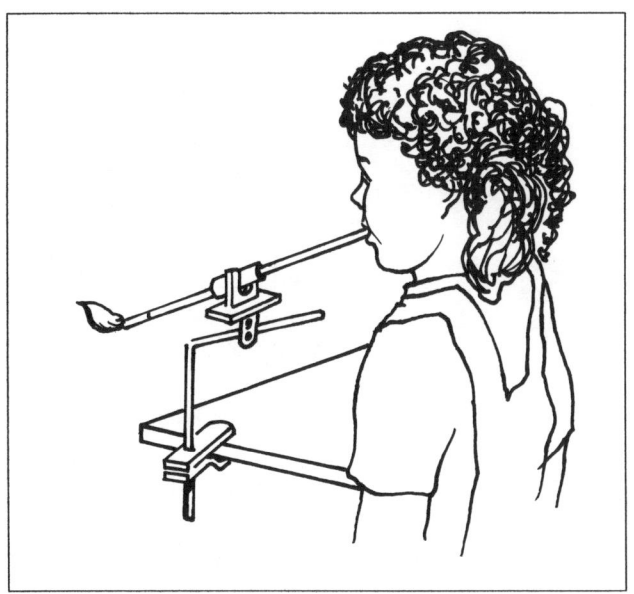

List seven types of adaptive equipment that can be used in pre-writing skills. What is the purpose of each?

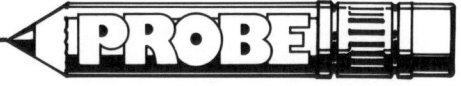

Distributors' Addresses

Adaptive Therapeutic Systems, Inc.
965 Dixwell Avenue
Hamden, CT 06514

Childcraft Education Corp.
20 Kilmer Road
P.O. Box 3081
Edison, NJ 08818-3081

Constructive Play Things
2008 West 103rd Terrace
Leawood, KS 66206

Help Yourself Aids
P.O. Box 192
Hinsdale, IL 60521

Ideal School Supply Company
11000 South Lavergne Avenue
Oak Lawn, IL 60453

Lakeshore Curriculum Materials
2695 East Dominguez Street
P.O. Box 6261
Carson, CA 90749

Medical Equipment Distributors
1701 South First Avenue
Maywood, IL 60153

Fred Sammons, Inc.
P.O. Box 32
Brookfield, IL 60513

Teaching Resources
50 Pond Park Road
Hingham, MA 02043

Teaching Tools
P.O. Box 27567
Phoenix, AZ 85061

Wayne Engineering
1825 West Willow Road
Northfield, IL 60093-2925

7 Movement and Pre-Writing Skills

Young children have a need to learn through movement experiences—exercises that utilize their large muscles and involve gross motor coordination. Numerous studies and experiments show that movement can positively affect learning. It can help reinforce the concept being taught and maintain the students' and teachers' interest level. And it's fun!

The movement activities given here can be used to reinforce the lines, circles, and other shapes being taught in pre-writing instruction. They can be modified as necessary for use with developmentally delayed children or adults.

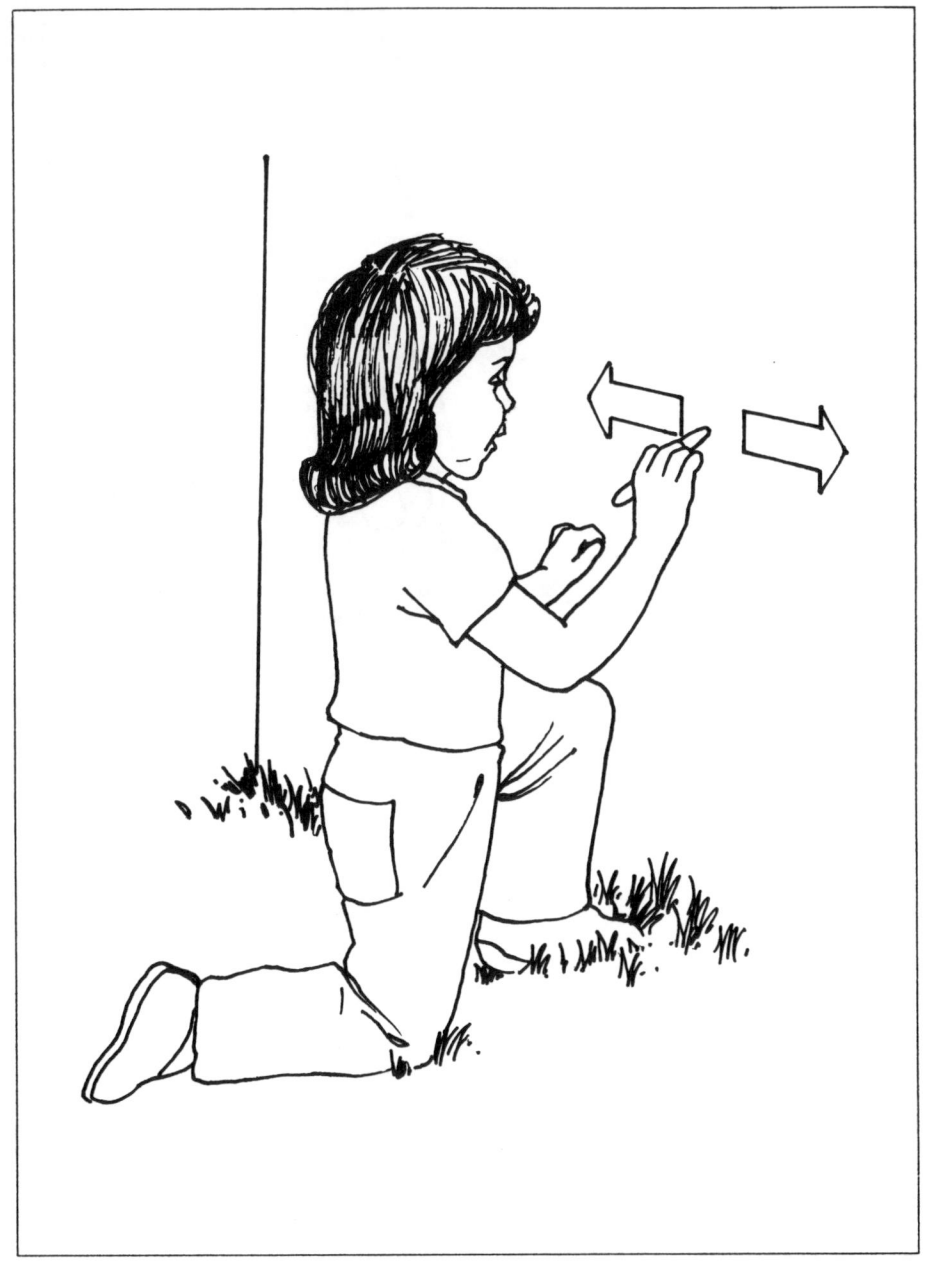

Activity 1   Have students walk on straight, curved, and diagonal lines.

— Have students walk on a board, a tape line, or a string line. They can walk with or without shoes.
— Have students help define the lines by placing a bean bag, ball, box, or toy at the beginning and end points. They can walk, run, crawl, or roll from the beginning to the end points.
— Have them walk on shapes drawn in sand.

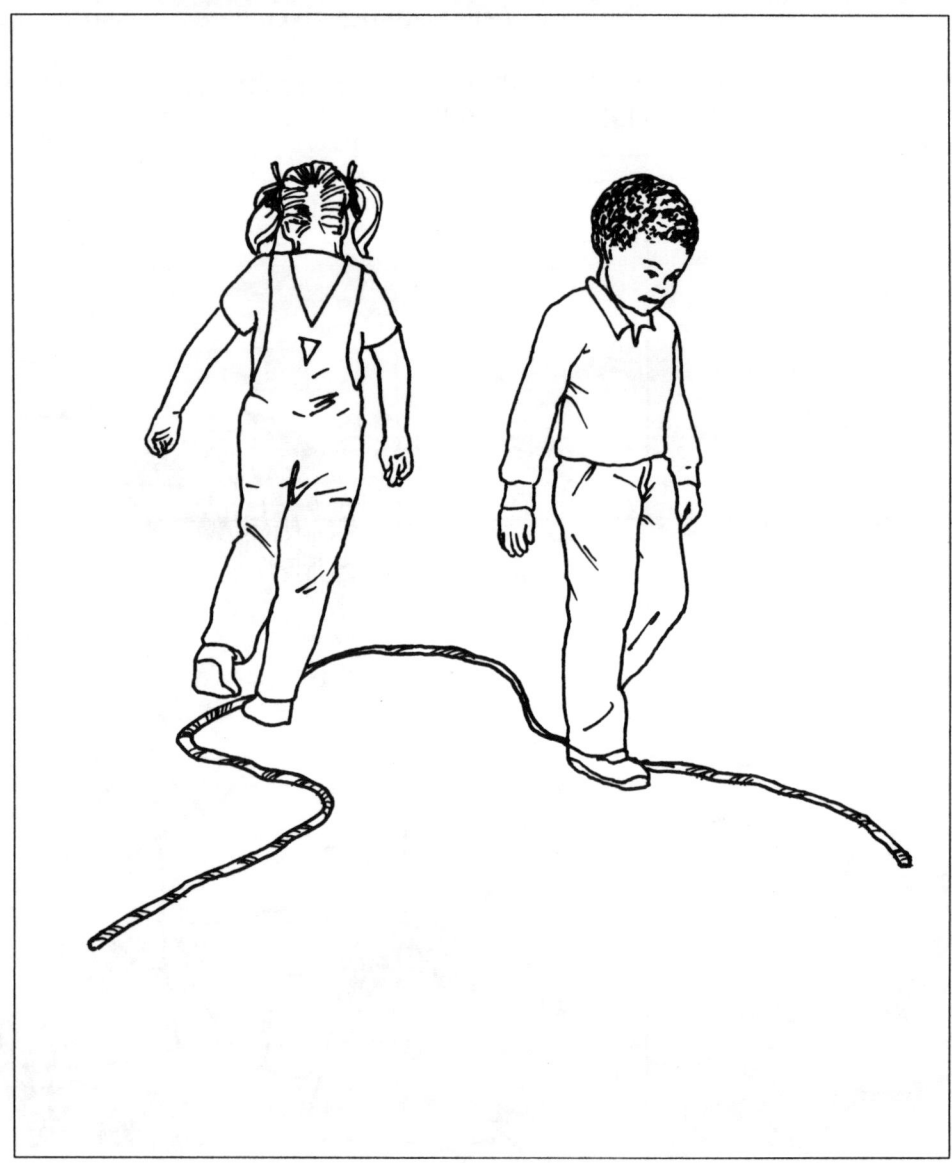

Activity 2 Have students walk, run, skip, crawl, creep, or knee-walk on a design on the floor.

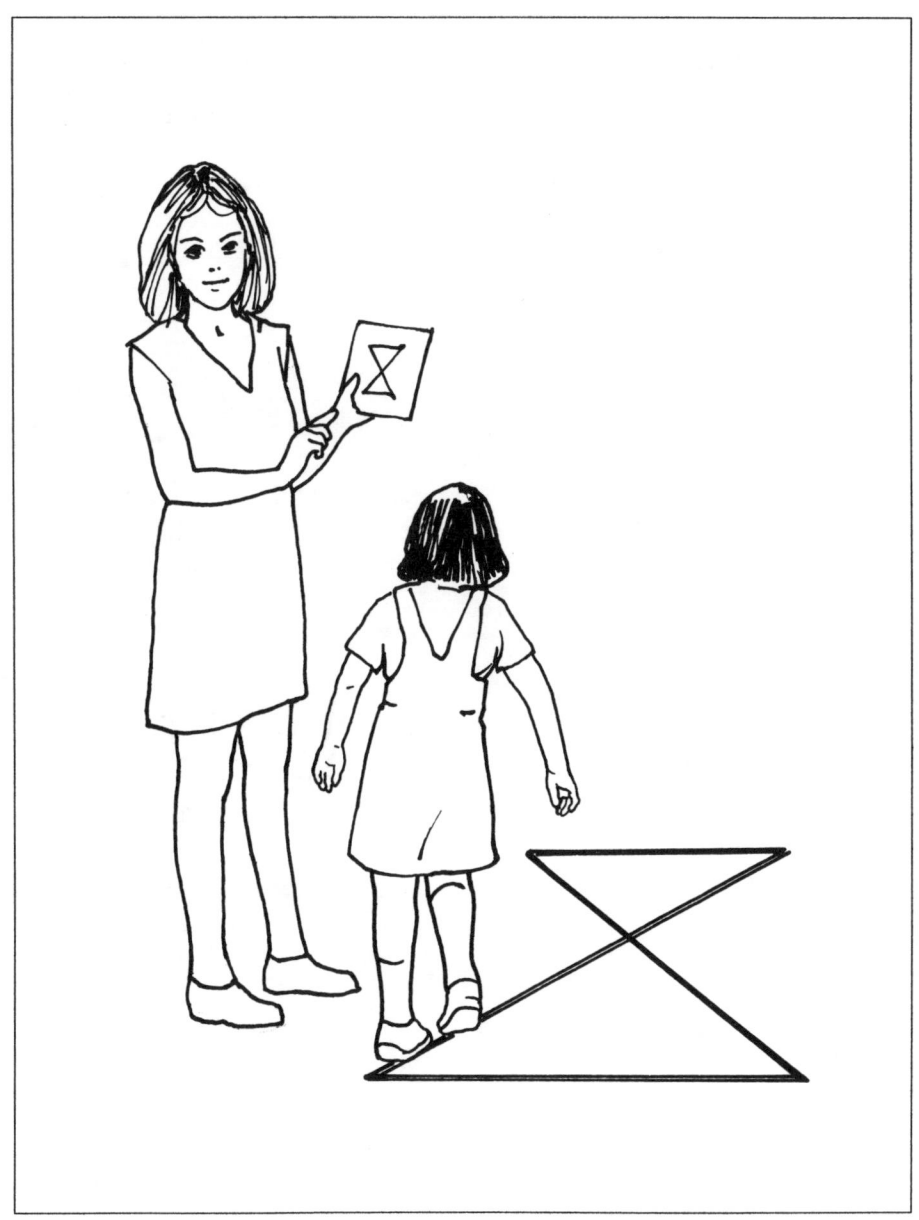

Activity 3 Have all the students join hands and make a circle. They can sing songs or play musical games in this position.

— Have them play Hokey Pokey in this circle position.
— Play Modified Musical Chairs, in which the students walk while the music is on and stop when the music stops.
— Play Pass the Hot Potato. Students pass an object rapidly around the circle until the music stops. Then, whoever has the "hot potato" is "out."

Activity 4 **Play Follow the Leader in different patterns.**
— Let the students take turns declaring the direction.

Activity 5 **Play hoop games to reinforce the concept of a circle.**
— Have the students feel around the hoop with their hands, arms, feet, or legs.
— Students can alternate having eyes open and eyes closed.

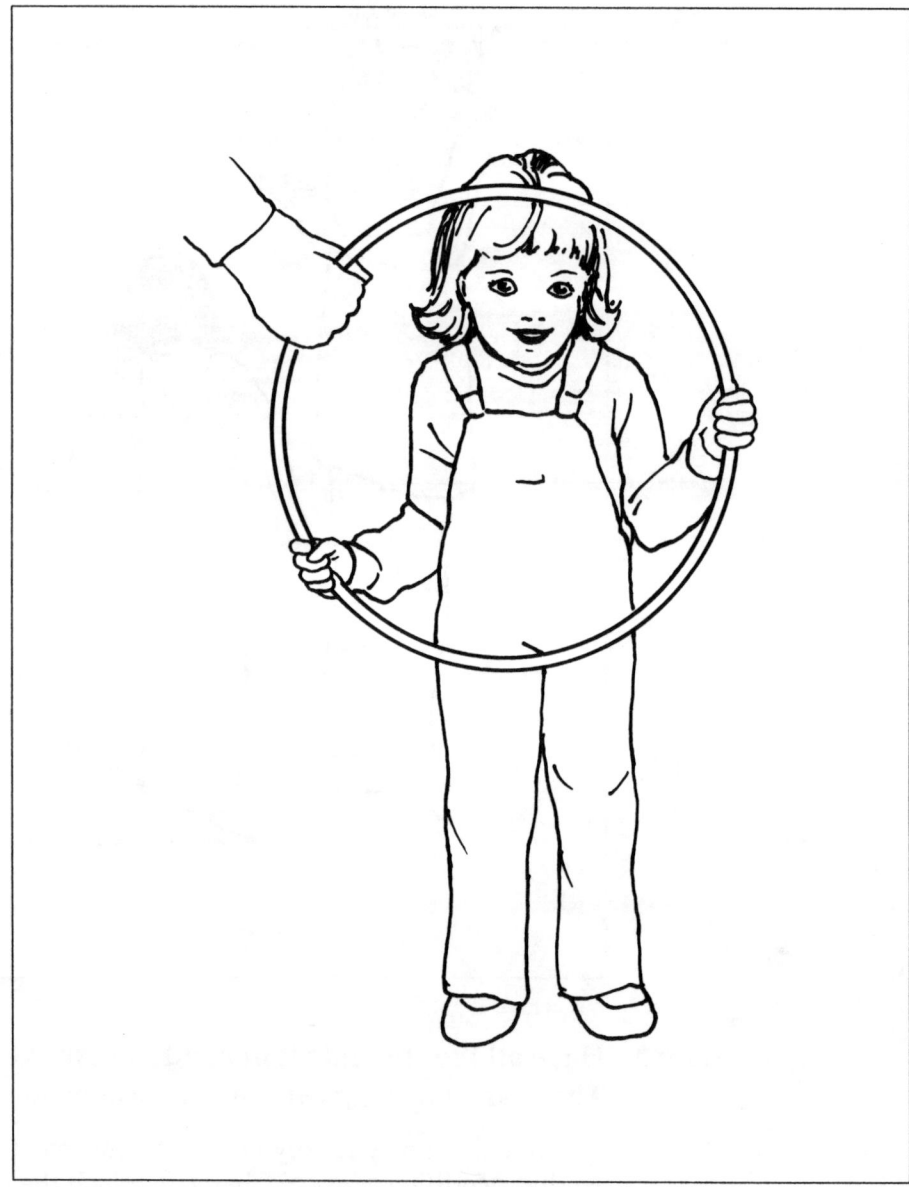

Activity 6 Play imitation games in which students form their bodies into a "line" (vertical, horizontal, or diagonal), a circle, or another shape.

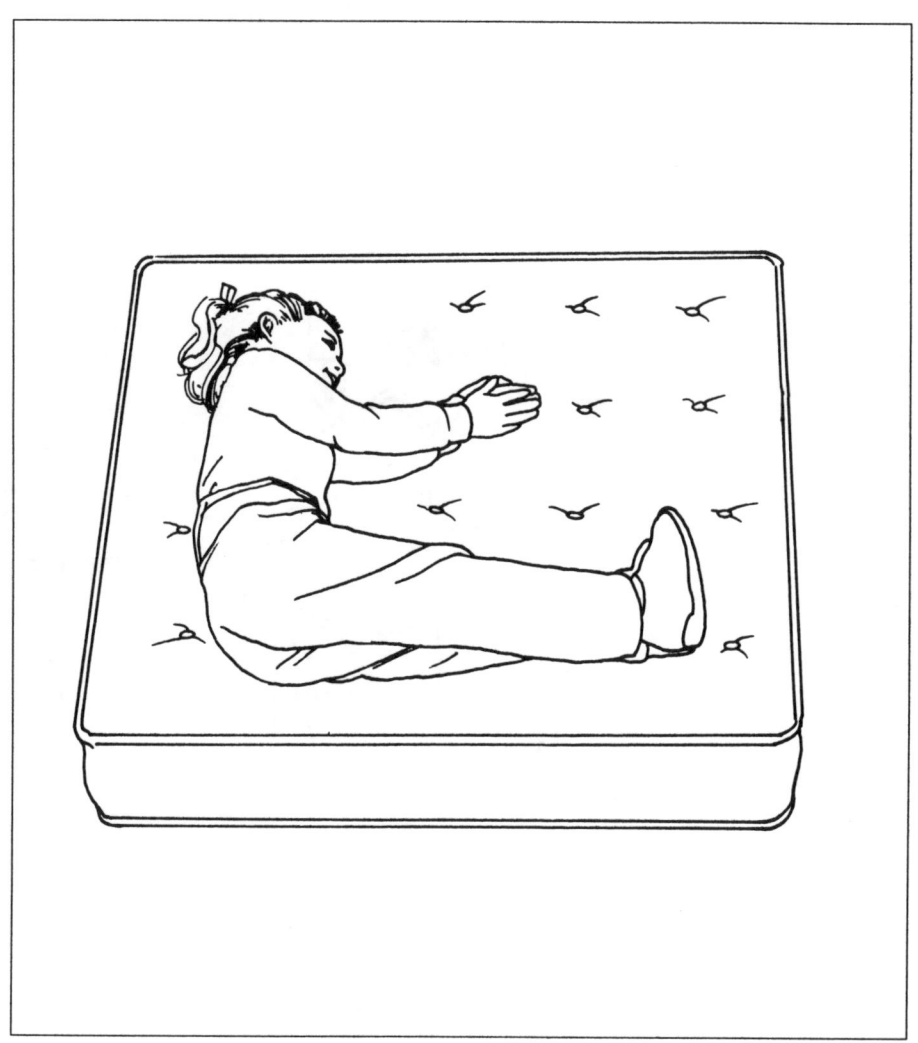

Activity 7 Have the students touch the edge of a square or round table while walking around it. Try this blindfolded or with vision.

— Tape a small reward on the side of the table, or place it on the surface. Let the children try to find the "treasure" while blindfolded.

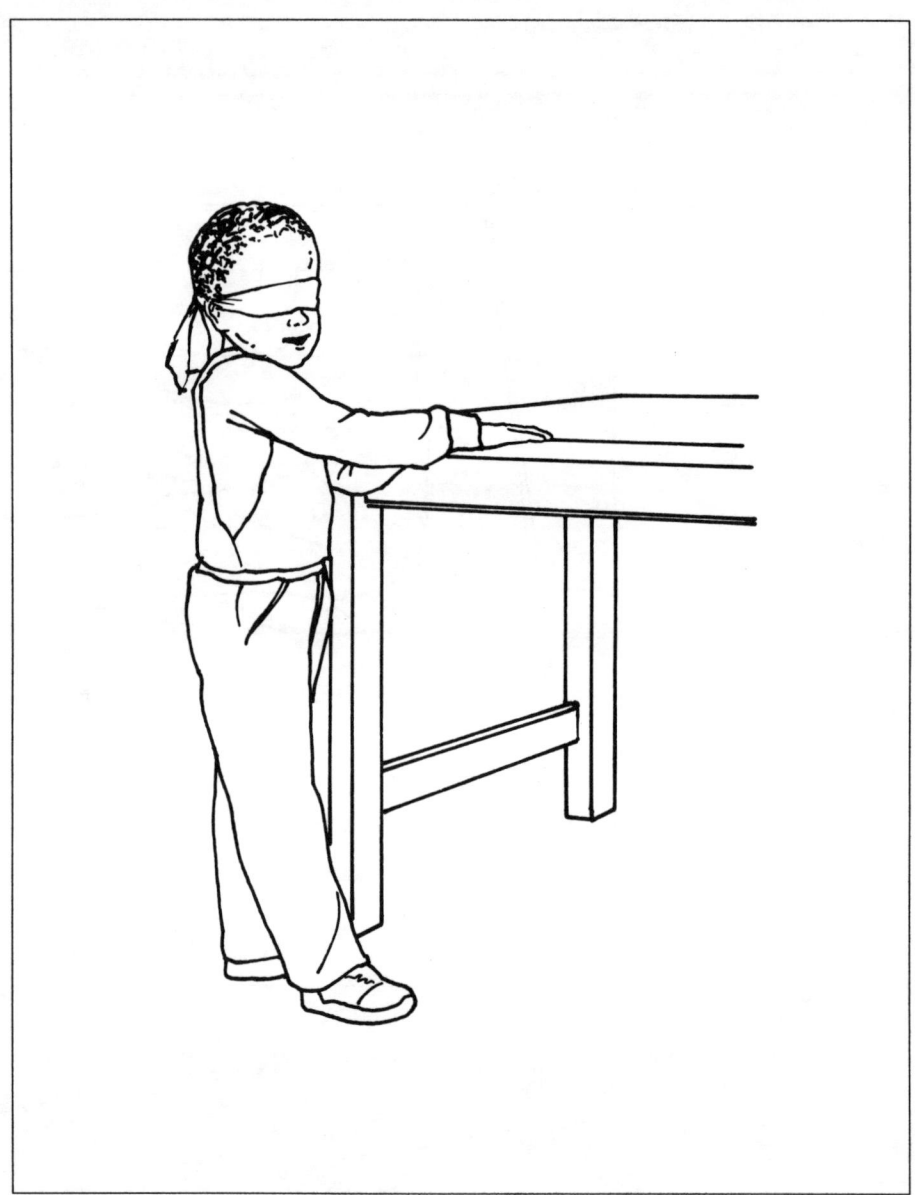

Describe seven movement activities that can be used to reinforce shapes important for pre-writing skills.

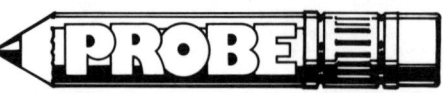

8 Pre-Writing Activities

The following activities are only a few that could be used to vary the teaching of pre-writing skills. They are meant to inspire your own thinking. At the end of the chapter, a blank activity sheet is included for your use. You may reproduce the form as often as you wish for recording your own ideas.

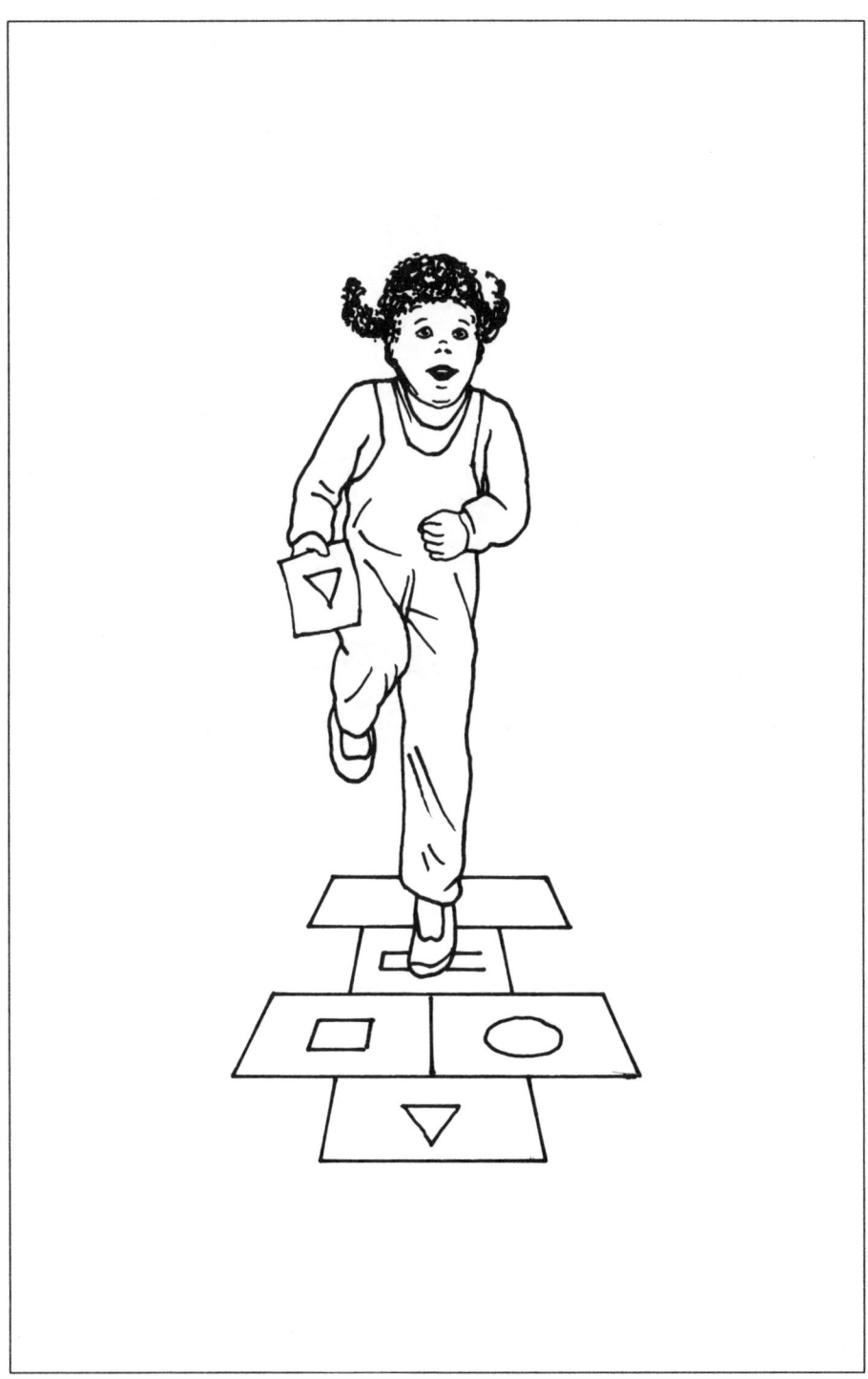

■ Finger Painting in the Bathtub

Purpose To give students preliminary pre-writing experience

Skill Stage Random scribbling or beginning of directional scribbling

Materials Ivory Snow Flakes finger paints (see recipe on page 44)

Position Sitting in the bathtub

Procedure Put the child in the bathtub with no water. Let the child finger paint all over the sides of the tub in any direction desired. Then turn on the water and wash the child and the tub.

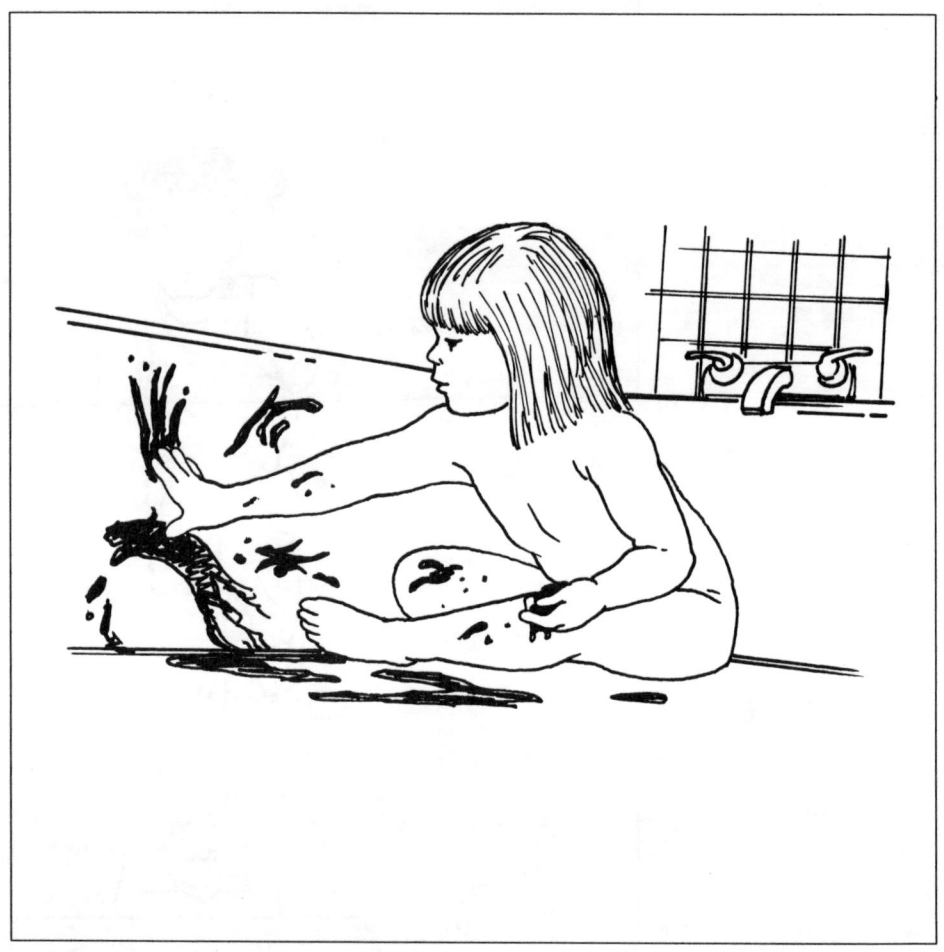

■ **Cornmeal Painting**

Purpose	To give students preliminary pre-writing experiences
Skill Stage	Random scribbling or beginning of directional scribbling
Materials	Cornmeal
Position	Standing, kneeling, or half-kneeling at a table
Procedure	Put a pile of cornmeal in front of each child. Let the children cover the table with cornmeal by finger painting with it.
Variations	Use dry oatmeal, lotions, whipped cream, puddings, or a combination of cornstarch and water.

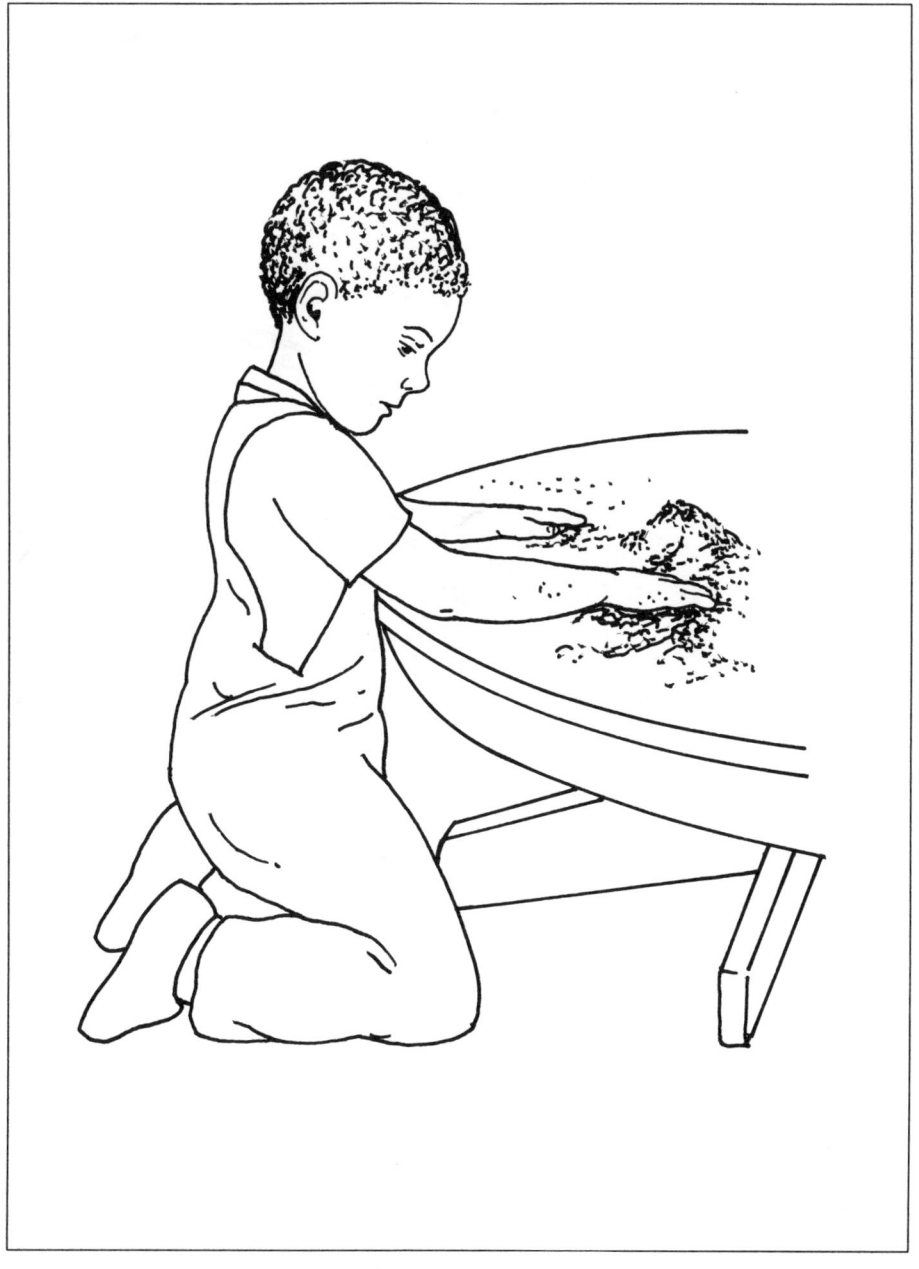

■ **Sand Drawing**

Purpose	To give students practice in imitating basic pre-writing shapes
Skill Stage	Imitation of basic shapes
Materials	Long sticks Sandbox or patch of sand
Position	Standing, kneeling, on all fours, half-kneeling, or walking outside
Procedure	Draw in the sand with a stick, and have the children imitate your shapes or scribbles in the sand. Let them hold the sticks with one or both hands to give experiences with both hands.
Variations	Have the students use toy rakes, shovels, brooms, or hoes to draw in the sand.

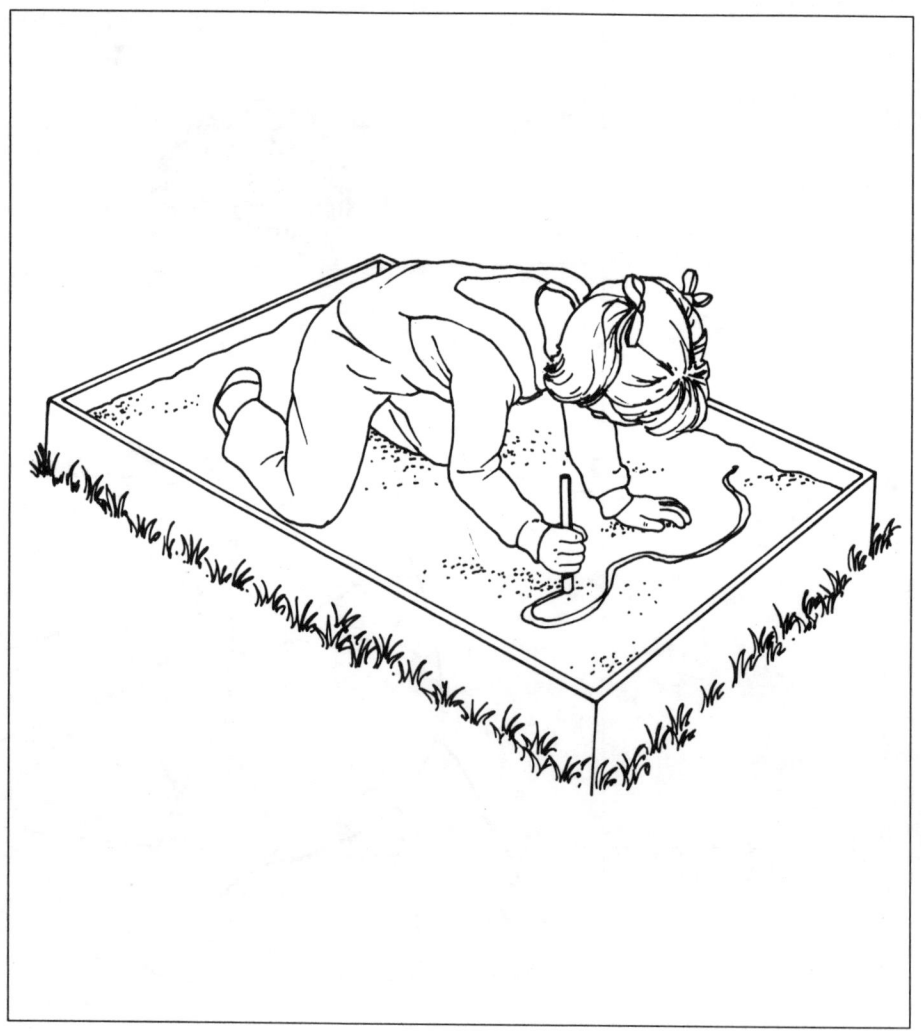

■ Water Painting

Purpose	To teach imitation of basic pre-writing skills
Skill Stage	Imitation of basic shapes
Materials	Wide and narrow paintbrushes Water
Position	Sitting, on all fours, kneeling, or squatting
Procedure	Go outside on a warm, dry day. Draw a scribble direction or line on the sidewalk with water. Have the children dip their paintbrushes in water and imitate or copy your scribble direction or line.

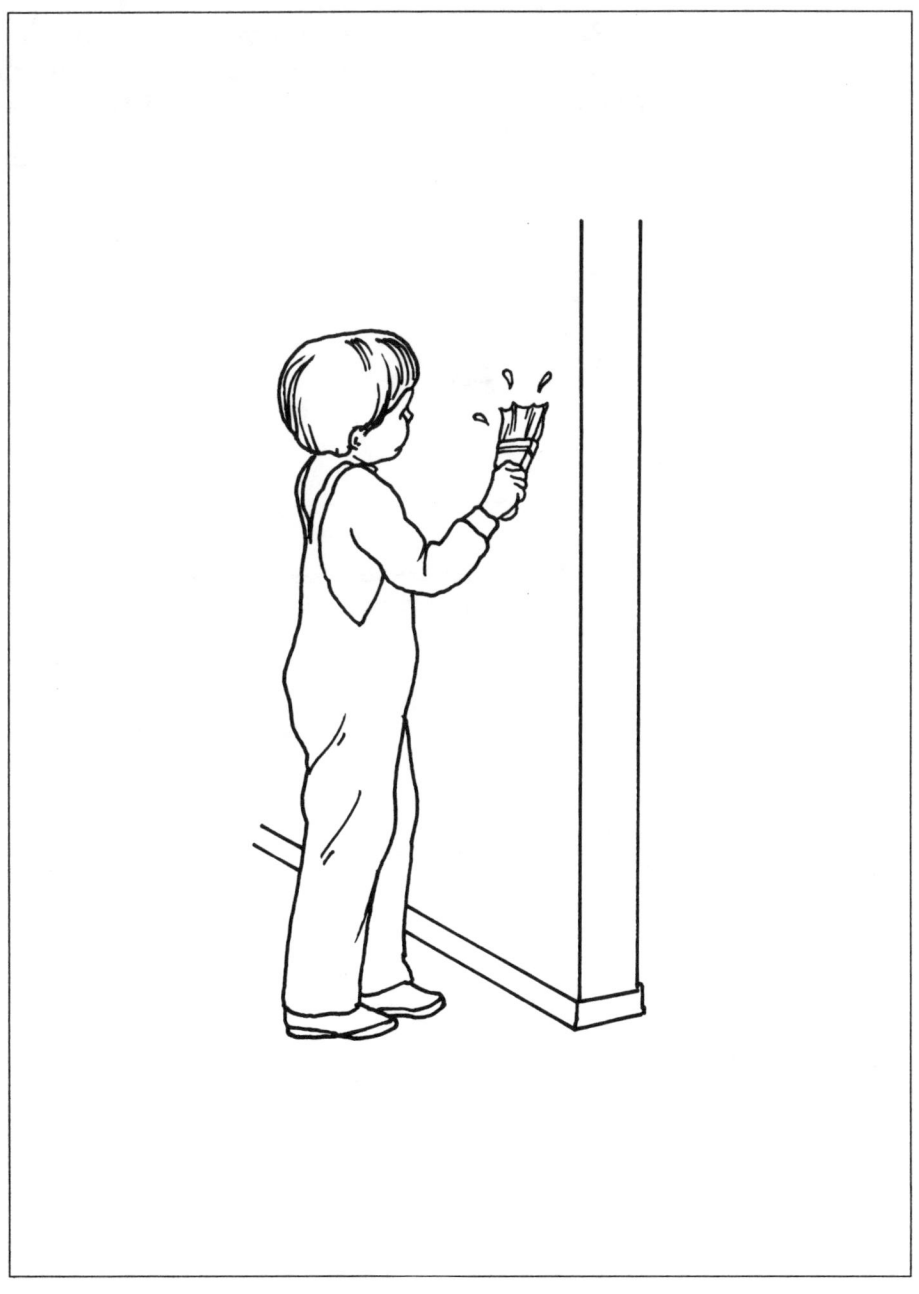

■ Stencil Drawing

Purpose	To teach imitation of basic pre-writing shapes
Skill Stage	Imitation of basic shapes
Materials	Stencils Crayons, markers, or finger paints
Position	Sitting, prone, kneeling, half-kneeling, on all fours, standing
Procedure	Give the students a stencil cut out of Plexiglas, cardboard, or fiberboard. Have them feel the shape with their fingers. Have them feel it again with their eyes closed. Then have them draw inside the stencil with crayons, markers, or finger paints. Remove the stencil so they can see what they have done. With the stencil removed, have them follow along the mark with a finger. Then have them try to repeat the shape without the stencil.
Variations	Stencils can be made of felt, sandpaper, or cloth of strong texture glued to a board.

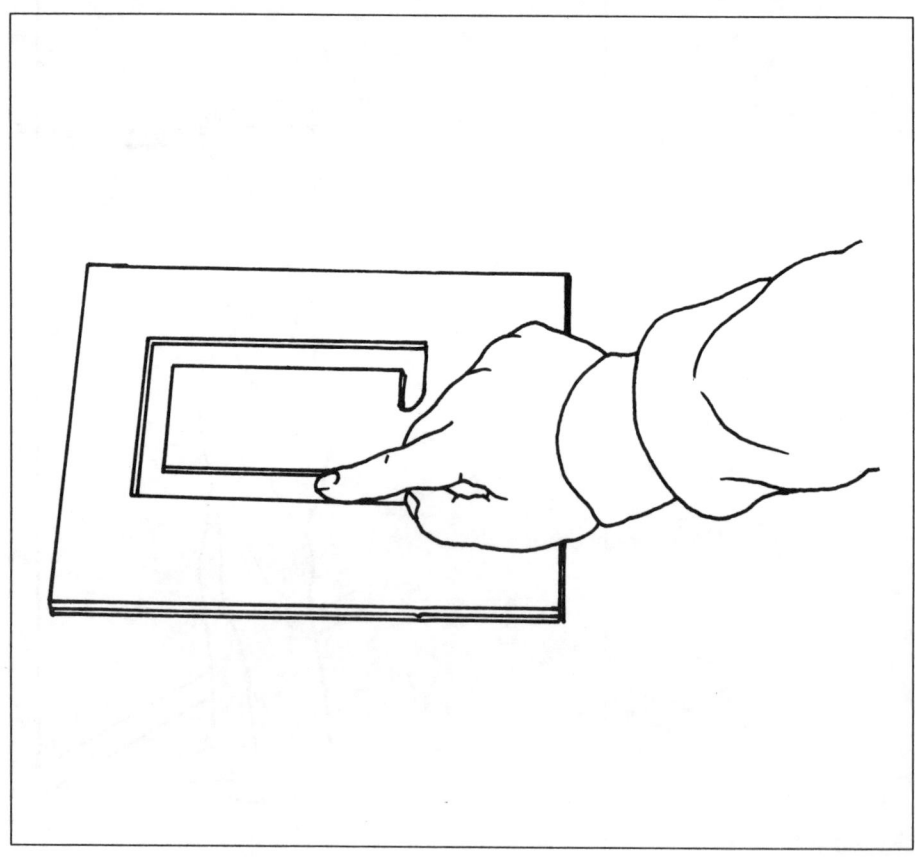

■ Circle Stopping

Purpose	To teach children to stop circular scribbling and draw circular lines
Skill Stage	Circle imitation
Materials	Marker Flat stick
Position	Sitting, prone, kneeling, half-kneeling, on all fours, standing
Procedure	Draw a large circle on a sheet of paper and place a flat stick at the beginning/ending point. Help the student to start at the beginning point, draw the circle, and *stop* at the flat stick instead of continuing as in scribbling.
Variations	Cut out a circular stencil in sandpaper and have the students use a flat stick. If the student goes outside the stencil line, immediate tactile feedback is given.

■ **Feely Shapes**

Purpose	To teach students to imitate pre-writing shapes
Skill Stage	Any level of line imitation
Materials	Cardboard Yarn, sandpaper, or flat sticks Finger paints or crayons
Position	Any position
Procedure	Make a specific shape on the cardboard with thick yarn, sandpaper, or flat sticks. Have the students feel the shape again and again with one or both hands. Then have them use finger paints or crayons to repeat the shape.
Variations	Try having the students do this activity blindfolded.

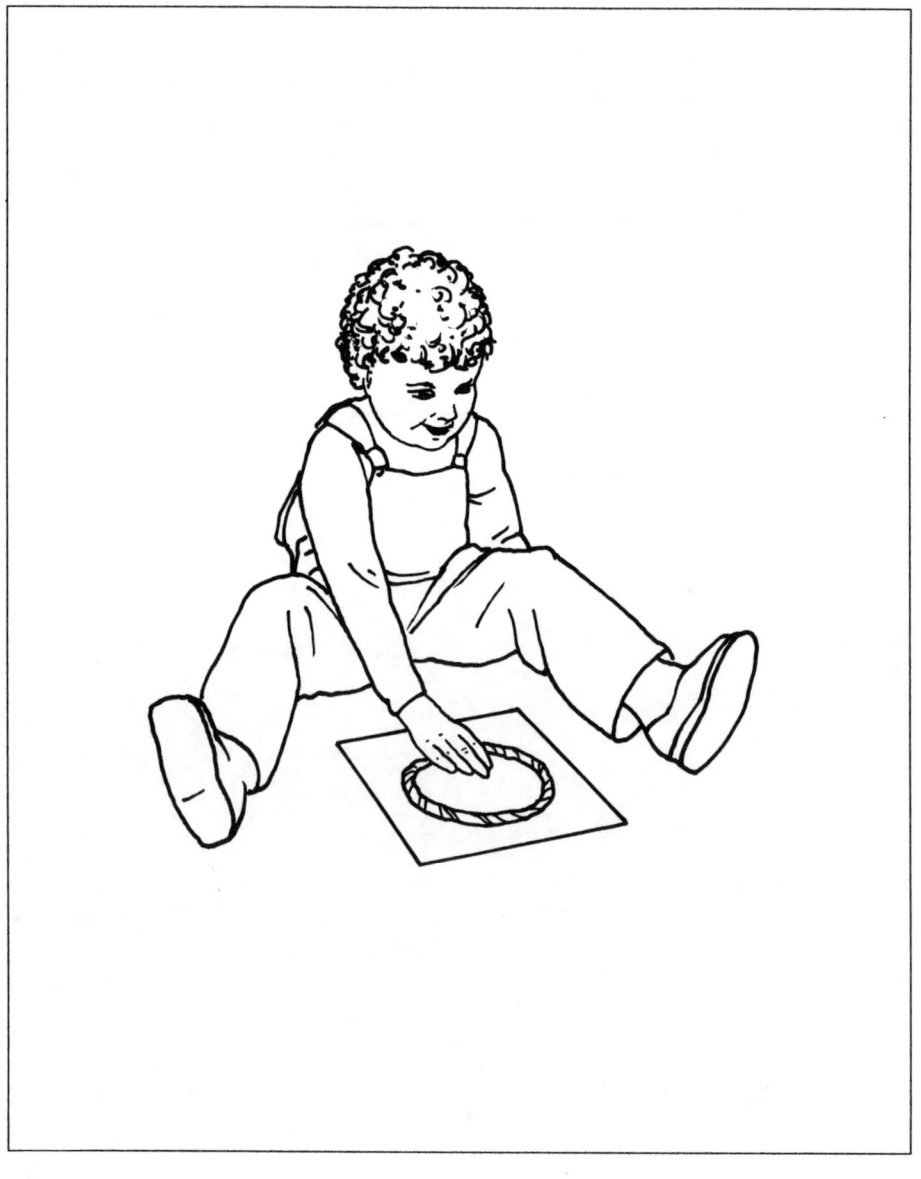

■ Racetrack Drawing

Purpose	To teach students to imitate or copy pre-writing shapes
Skill Stage	Imitation of scribbling or any level of line
Materials	Sand Toy cars
Position	Any position
Procedure	Make a "racetrack" in the sand, using any of the pre-writing shapes. Let the students run the cars back and forth in the shape or around the shape.
Variations	Have the students race their cars on racetracks drawn in the sand or on tracks made in or through sandpaper or between two strings or yarn pieces.

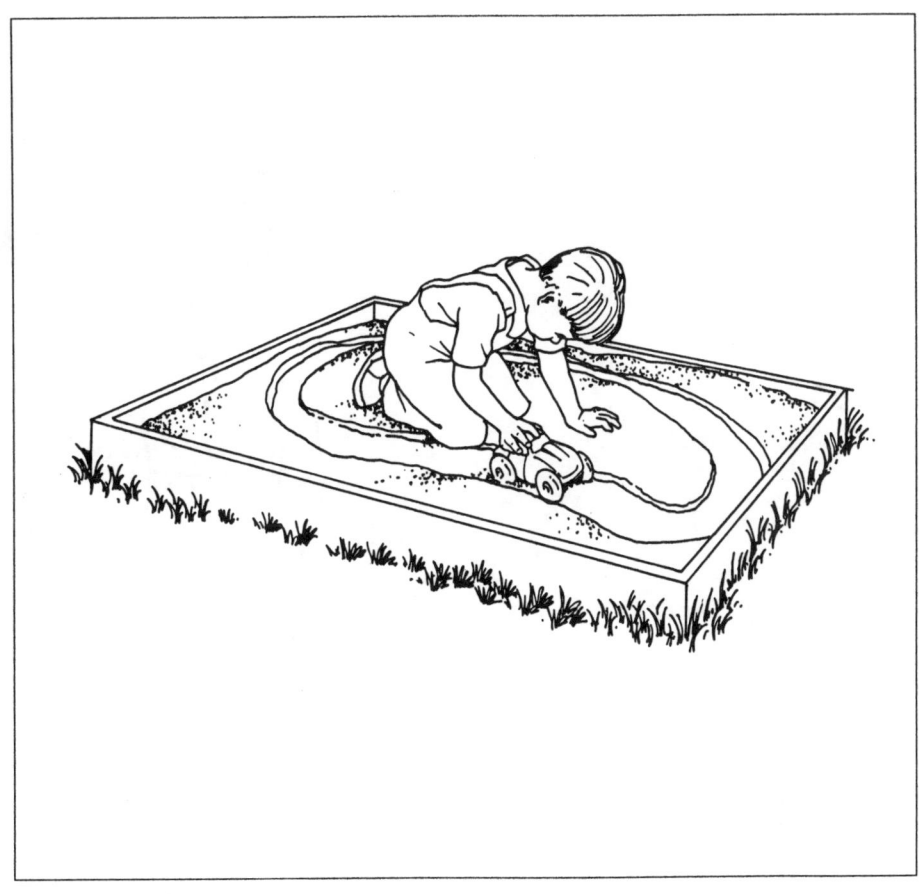

■ Table-Wipe Drawing

Purpose	To teach beginning pre-writing scribble imitation
Skill Stage	Vertical, horizontal, or circular scribble imitation
Materials	Washcloth Table
Position	Standing
Procedure	Have the students imitate wiping the table up and down, back and forth, or in a circular direction. You do it, then have the students do it.
Variations	Have the student wipe a low chalkboard with an eraser or wipe a window with cloths and cleaner in a particular scribble direction.

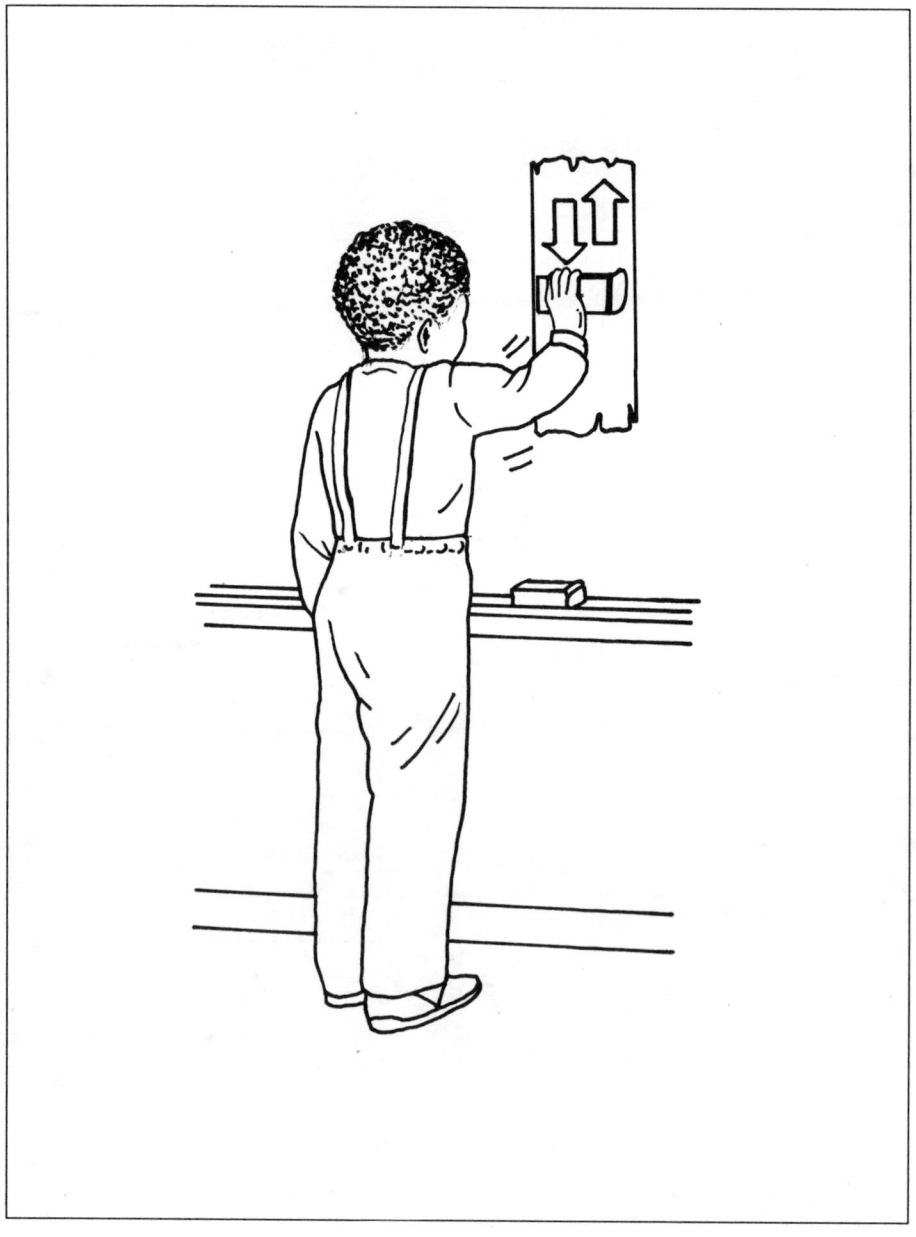

■ Star Tracking

Purpose	To teach students to imitate pre-writing shapes
Skill Stage	Imitation of any pre-writing shape
Materials	Paper Gummed stars
Position	Any position
Procedure	Paste stars on a paper at the beginning, end, or corners of a shape. Have the students draw from star to star to make the shape. Then have them draw the shape without the stars.
Variations	Punch holes in paper to make a shape. Then have the students draw from one punched hole to another.

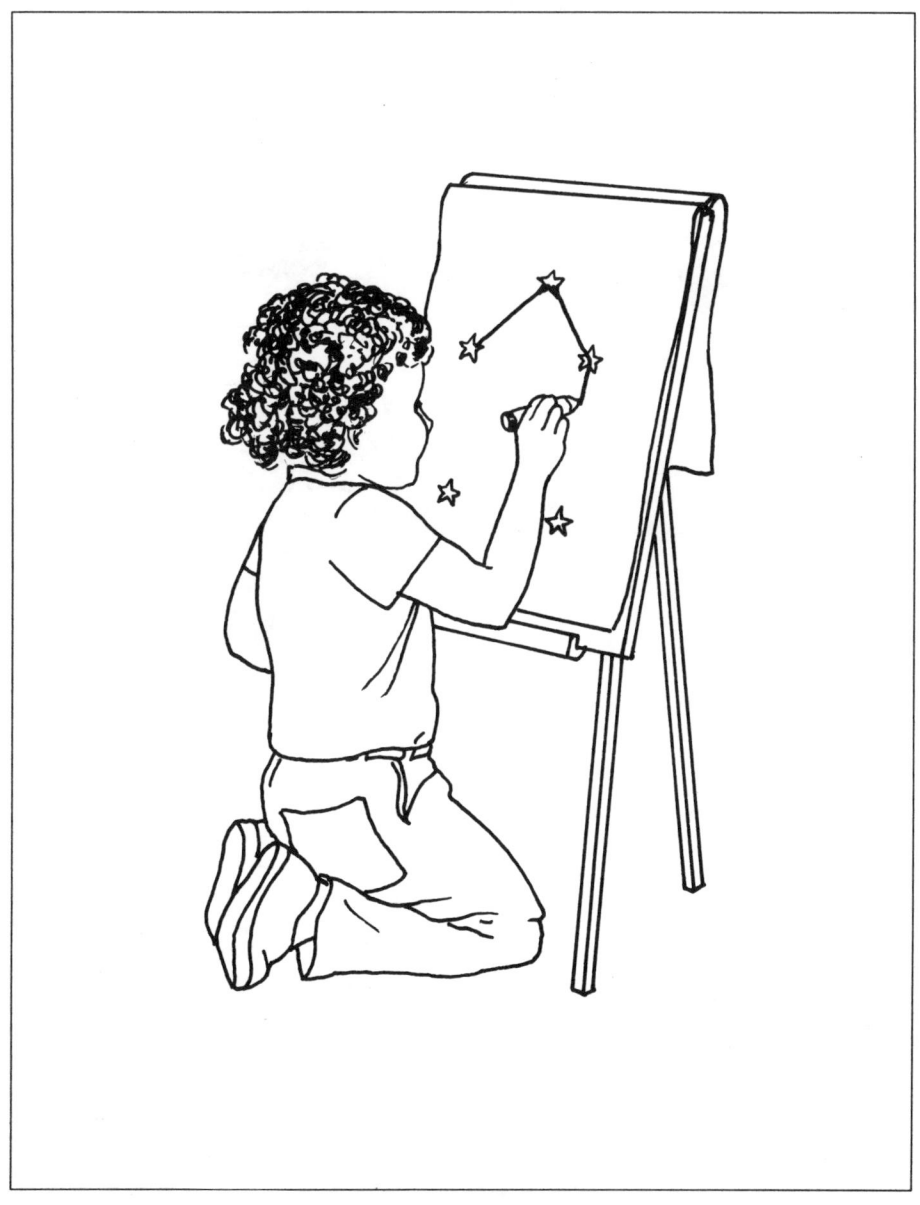

■ **Sand Shapes**

Purpose	To teach students to imitate or copy pre-writing shapes
Skill Stage	Imitation of any shapes
Materials	Sand
Position	Sitting
Procedure	Have the students imitate or copy a shape by drawing in the sand with a foot. Help them keep their balance during the movement, as needed.
Variations	Have the students try to draw with their elbows or one finger.

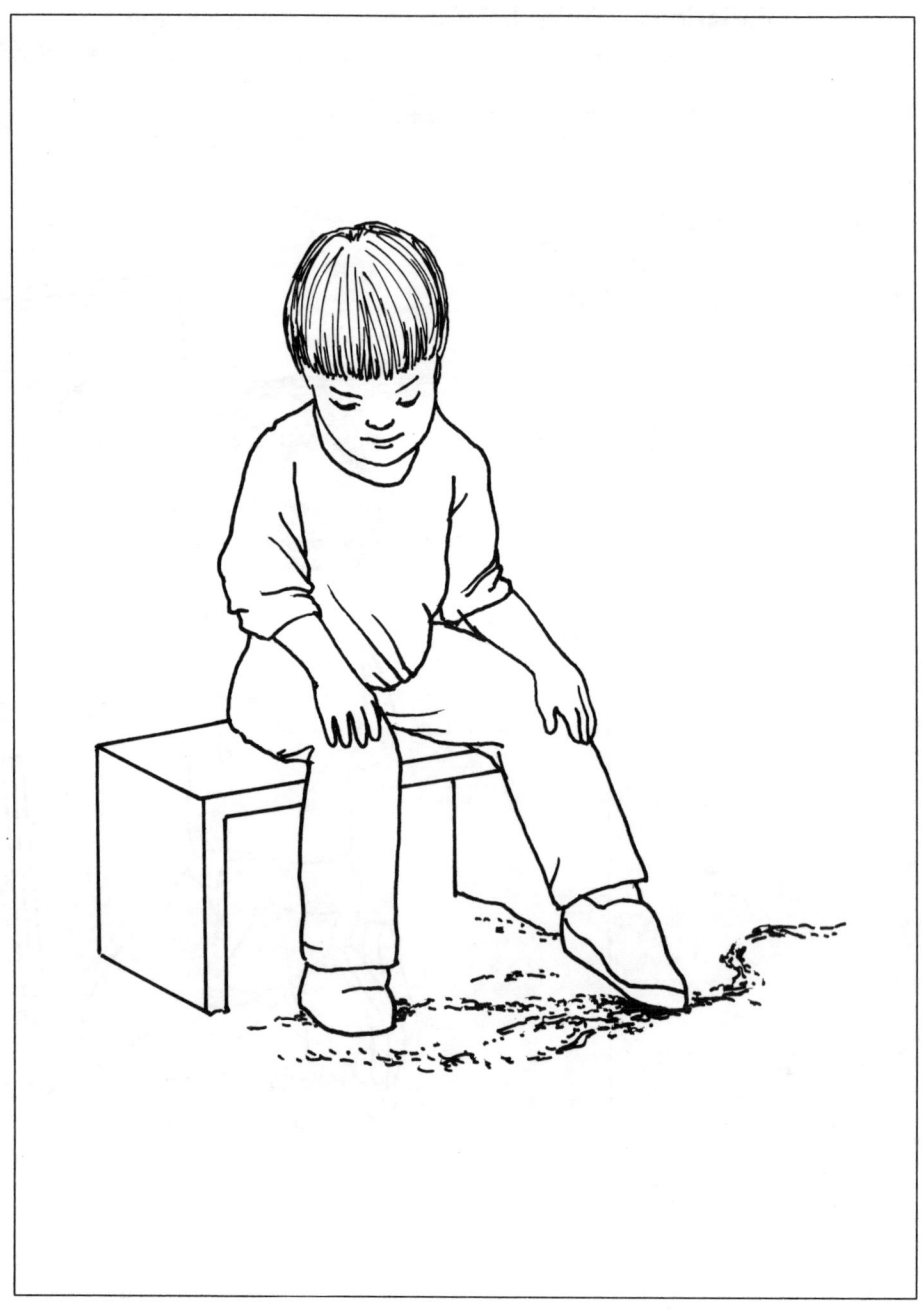

■ Simon Sez

Purpose   To teach imitation of basic pre-writing shapes

Skill Stage   Imitation of basic shapes

Materials   None

Position   All positions

Procedure   Play Simon Sez with a group of students, making their movements reinforce the basic pre-writing shapes. For example, have the children make pointers with fingers interlocked and move them up and down, back and forth, or in a circle.

Variations   Imitative movements can be incorporated into many children's song games (The People on the Bus, Hokey Pokey, and others).

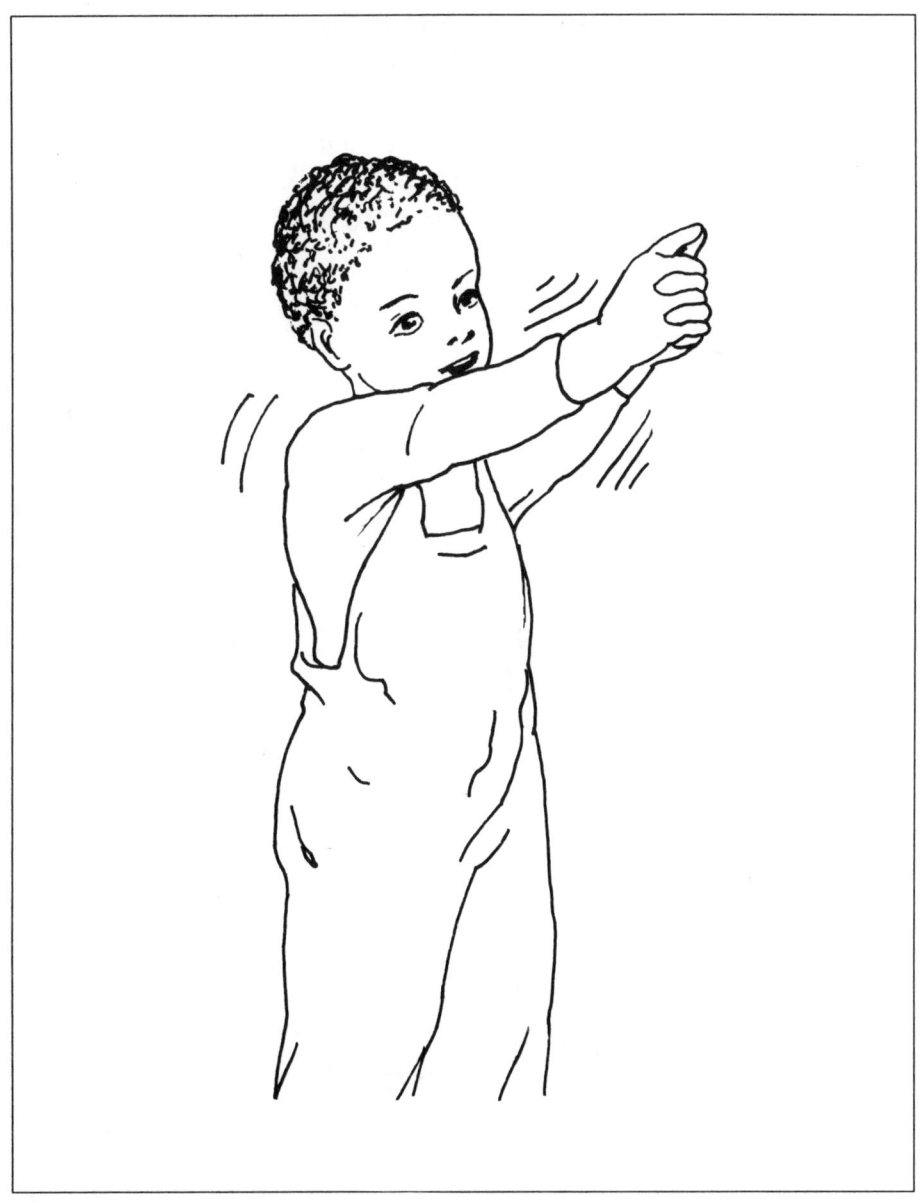

■ Drawing in the Air

Purpose	To teach students to imitate or copy vertical, horizontal, or circular scribble movement, using gross motor activity
Skill Stage	Imitation of basic pre-writing shapes
Materials	An empty paper-towel roll Crepe-paper streamers or cut-out paper stars
Position	Standing, kneeling, or half-kneeling
Procedure	Attach crepe-paper streamers or stars to the end of the paper-towel roll to make a "magic wand." Stand facing or next to the children. Alternate holding the wand with both hands or either hand. Wave the wand in the air in a vertical, horizontal, or circular direction. Have the student imitate the movement. Reverse the lead so that sometimes you are imitating the students and sometimes they are imitating you.
Variations	1. "Draw" shapes or letters in the air. 2. Combine sounds with the movements. 3. Have the children walk while doing the imitation. This makes the movement more difficult.

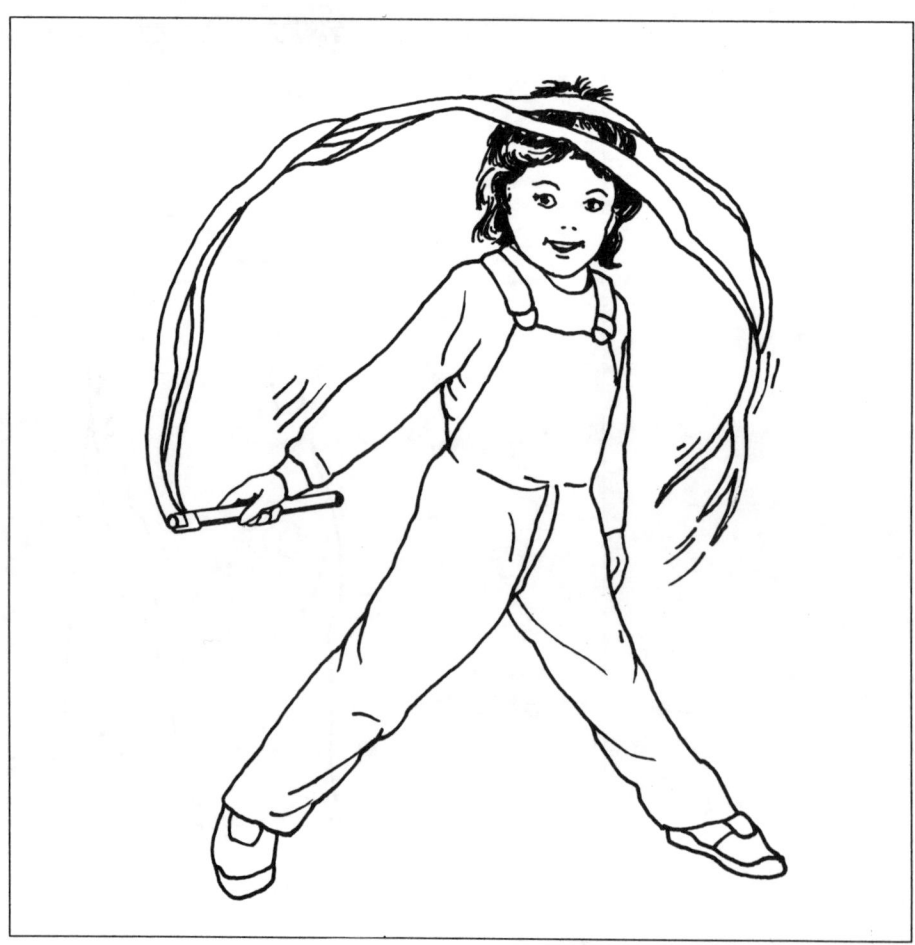

■ Sandbox Drawing

Purpose	To teach students to imitate a circular line and to increase tactile awareness
Skill Stage	Imitation of circle
Materials	Cardboard box Sand Stick
Position	Standing, kneeling, or half-kneeling
Procedure	Cut the cardboard box so the edges are 2 inches to 4 inches high. Fill it with sand. Help the students to draw a circle with a stick or finger. Then have them use the stick or finger to trace the circle.
Variations	1. Wet the sand for increased resistance. 2. Race a toy truck around a track drawn in the sand.

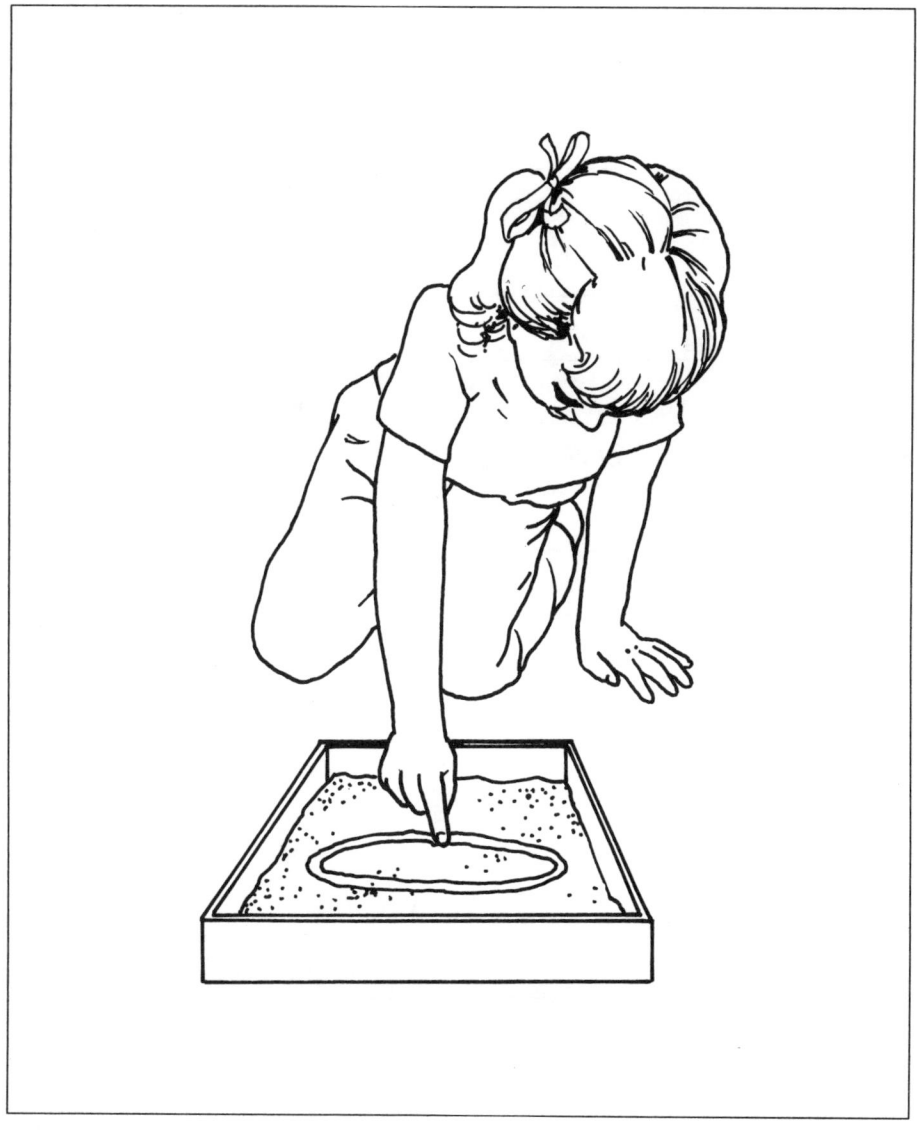

Pre-Writing Activity

Purpose _____
_____

Skill Stage _____
_____

Materials _____
_____
_____
_____
_____

Position _____
_____

Procedure _____
_____
_____
_____
_____
_____
_____
_____

Variation _____
_____
_____
_____
_____

© 1990 by Communication Skill Builders, Inc.
This page may be reproduced for instructional use.

9 Weekly Activity Planning

Now you know how to assess pre-writing skills and choose a progression of goals. You've read about different pre-writing materials that stimulate various sensory channels, different positions in which to do pre-writing tasks, and different ways to incorporate movement into the instruction. Now you can plan individualized pre-writing programs for each of your students.

Use the reproducible Weekly Pre-Writing Activity Plan form on the following page to plan individualized activities that will be varied and fun. A sample week of activities for a student is given on page 107.

Choose a pre-writing skill stage of development, and think of how many ways you can teach that behavior.

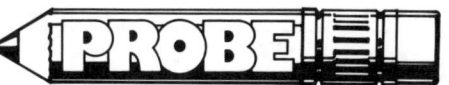

Weekly Pre-Writing Activity Plan

Student _____

Week _____

Objective _____

_____

DAY	ACTIVITY	POSITION	MOVEMENT
Monday			
Tuesday			
Wednesday			
Thursday			
Friday			

© 1990 by Communication Skill Builders, Inc.
This page may be reproduced for administrative use.

Sample
Weekly Pre-Writing Activity Plan

Student_____

Week_____

Objective_____

_____

DAY	ACTIVITY	POSITION	MOVEMENT
Monday	Draw in sand with a car or stick	All fours	Creep to the sandbox
Tuesday	Feel a yarn circle or a sandpaper circle	Kneeling, standing, or marching	Play games in circles with other children
Wednesday	Draw in air with a paper-towel roll "wand"	Standing	Walk from station to station, draw in air, move to next station
Thursday	Finger paint with scented paint	Prone	Roll to the finger-paint station
Friday	Draw with a weighted paintbrush	Half-kneeling or standing at an easel	Hop to the easel

10 Planning an Individual Pre-Writing Program

The next step is to set up a long-range learning plan for the individual student or students with whom you are concerned. Whether you develop an informal program or a formal written program to meet your federal, state, or local standards, the following should be considered:

1. Learner's developmental pre-writing skills
2. Long-term goal
3. Sequential objective
4. Equipment and materials
5. Position
6. Environment
7. Methodology
8. Maintenance activities

Here are some suggestions on each specific factor in the individual pre-writing program.

1 Developmental Pre-Writing Skills

What is the learner's current level of performance? At what stage does the pre-writing checklist show the student to be succeeding? Clearly indicate what the learner can and cannot do in pre-writing tasks. Are there any motoric or sensory limitations that affect pre-writing skills?

2 Long-Term Goal

What is a realistic long-term expectation for this learner? Do you expect total independence in writing, or is simply learning to write an adapted (simplified) signature or learning to use an adaptive writing tool such as a computer or a typewriter more realistic for this learner?

3 Sequential Objective

What is the specific next behavior to be learned? Is this sequential objective learnable? Is it broken down into small enough steps so that the student can succeed? Is the objective written in behavioral terms that can be measured? What is the criterion for success? How often does the task need to be performed successfully before the student should advance to the next step? It is important to write this objective specifically in order to document progress and help the student succeed.

4 Equipment and Materials

What materials will be used to maximize the sensory information presented? How many ways can the same objective be taught, using different media for the same outcome? Are adaptive writing tools needed for immediate or long-term success? Is a special weighted or adapted pencil needed? Will the adaptive materials be phased out, or are they long-term? Be sure to try a variety of equipment and materials and choose the most successful tools.

5 Position

What position will be used to teach this pre-writing skill? What position will be used to practice it? How can movement be incorporated into the instruction of this skill?

6 Environment

Where will the student sit or be positioned when performing this task? Are there any special considerations imposed by the person's physical limitations? Are there distractions to be minimized?

7 Methodology

How are you going to teach this behavior? Any task analysis should include the following components:

As a teacher, what will you do or say to elicit the response?

What is the learner expected to do or say in response?

What type of reinforcement will be provided for correct response?

What action will the teacher take if the learner responds incorrectly to the original directions? (Repeat directions? Provide an imitative model? Provide physical assistance?)

How will the data be collected?

8 Maintenance Activities

What activities will the student practice to ensure that the learned behavior is maintained? It is important to provide the student with the opportunity to practice this newly learned skill so that the behavior is maintained.

Individual Pre-Writing Program

Name_____

Classroom_____Date_____

Developmental Pre-Writing Skills _____
_____
_____

Long-Term Goal _____
_____
_____

Sequential Objective _____
_____
_____

Equipment and Materials _____
_____
_____

Position _____
_____
_____

Environment _____
_____
_____

Methodology _____
_____

Maintenance Activities _____
_____
_____
_____
_____
_____
_____

© 1990 by Communication Skill Builders, Inc.
This page may be reproduced for administrative use.

Post-Test

A. List nine prerequisite skills for pre-writing.
   1. _____
   2. _____
   3. _____
   4. _____
   5. _____
   6. _____
   7. _____
   8. _____
   9. _____

B. What is the difference between imitation and copying?
   _____
   _____
   _____
   _____
   _____
   _____

C. What is the developmental sequence of acquiring pre-writing skills?
   1. _____
   2. _____
   3. _____
   4. a. _____
      b. _____
   5. _____
   6. a. _____
      b. _____
      c. _____
   7. a. _____
      b. _____
      c. _____
   8. a. _____
      b. _____

9. a.___
   b.___
10. a.___
    b.___
11. a.___
    b.___
12. a.___
    b.___
13. a.___
    b.___
14. a.___
    b.___
15. a.___
    b.___
16. ___

D. What is the developmental sequence of learning to color a picture area?
   1. ___
   2. ___
   3. ___
   4. ___
   5. ___
   6. ___

E. What is the developmental sequence of learning stroke control in coloring?
   1. ___
   2. ___
   3. ___
   4. ___

F. What is the developmental sequence of learning to use color?
   1. ___
   2. ___
   3. ___
   4. ___

G. Name two visual media that can be used in choosing pre-writing materials.
   1. _____
   2. _____

H. Name two tactile media that can be used in choosing pre-writing materials.
   1. _____
   2. _____

I. Name two olfactory media that can be used in choosing pre-writing materials.
   1. _____
   2. _____

J. Name two auditory media that can be used in choosing pre-writing materials.
   1. _____
   2. _____

K. Name two gustatory media that can be used in choosing pre-writing materials.
   1. _____
   2. _____

L. Name two proprioceptive media that can be used in choosing pre-writing materials.
   1. _____
   2. _____

M. Describe a stable seating option, tell when it is used, and name two stable seating options.
   1. _____
   2. _____

N. Describe a practice seating option, tell when it is used, and name five practice seating options.
   1. _____
   2. _____
   3. _____
   4. _____
   5. _____

O. Name five things that can be done to improve stability for pre-writing functions.
   1. _____
   2. _____
   3. _____
   4. _____
   5. _____

P. Describe how the use of tools influences development of hand dominance.
   _____
   _____
   _____

Q. Name an activity that can assist the writer who has poor two-hand usage.
   _____
   _____
   _____

R. For each of the following categories, list a pre-writing activity that does not require usual writing tools.
   1. Gross motor activities_____
   2. Fine motor activities_____
   3. Sensory activities_____
   4. Daily living activities_____

S. Name two options that may assist in moving from an immature to a mature grasp.
   1. _____
   2. _____

T. List six ways to vary sensory aspects of the pre-writing task to help students improve their attention span.
   1. _____
   2. _____
   3. _____
   4. _____
   5. _____
   6. _____

© 1990 by Communication Skill Builders, Inc.
This page may be reproduced for administrative use.

U. Describe two ways to increase sensory information in an imitation activity.
   1. _____
   2. _____

V. Describe two ways to provide sensory information for children with limited vision.
   1. _____
   2. _____

W. Name two ways for students to practice pre-writing concepts when they do not have functional use of their hands.

   _____
   _____
   _____
   _____
   _____
   _____
   _____

X. List seven types of adaptive equipment that can be used in teaching pre-writing skills, and explain the purpose of each.
   1. _____
   2. _____
   3. _____
   4. _____
   5. _____
   6. _____
   7. _____

Y. List seven movement activities that can be used to reinforce shapes important for pre-writing skills.
   1. _____
   2. _____
   3. _____
   4. _____
   5. _____
   6. _____
   7. _____

Z. List five classroom activities that can be used to teach pre-writing skills.

1. _____
2. _____
3. _____
4. _____
5. _____

AA. Describe how the same pre-writing activity can be taught in a variety of ways.

_____
_____
_____
_____
_____
_____
_____
_____
_____

BB. Describe how to incorporate information about pre-writing skills into an Individual Pre-Writing Program.

_____
_____
_____
_____
_____
_____
_____
_____
_____
_____
_____
_____
_____
_____
_____
_____

© 1990 by Communication Skill Builders, Inc.
This page may be reproduced for administrative use.

Readings

Banus, B. *The developmental therapist: A prototype of the pediatric occupational therapist.* Thorofare, N.J.: Charles B. Slack, 1971.

Cratty, B. *Active learning.* Englewood Cliffs, N.J.: Prentice-Hall, Inc., 1971.

Dunaway, A., and M. D. Klein. *Writing techniques and adaptations for home and classroom.* Tucson, Ariz.: Communication Skill Builders, 1988.

Harnstock, E. *Teaching Montessori in the home: The pre-school years.* New York: Random House, 1968.

Kephart, N. *The slow learner in the classroom.* Columbus, Ohio: Charles E. Merrill Publishing Company, 1960.

Olsen, J. Z. *Handwriting without tears.* Brookfield, Ill.: Fred Sammons, Inc., 1980.